SOCIOLOGY
AND THE FIELD OF
PUBLIC HEALTH

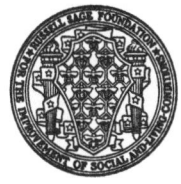

*Prepared for the
American Sociological Association*
By EDWARD A. SUCHMAN
Professor of Sociology
University of Pittsburgh

RUSSELL SAGE FOUNDATION
New York   1963

© 1963
RUSSELL SAGE FOUNDATION
Printed in the United States
  of America

Printed November, 1963
Reprinted June, 1966
Reprinted April, 1968

*Library of Congress
Catalog Card Number: 63-21228*

WM. F. FELL CO., PRINTERS
PHILADELPHIA, PA.

To the Memory
of
My Mother

CONTENTS

Foreword by Leonard S. Cottrell, Jr.	5
Acknowledgments	7
I. Introduction	9
II. The Growth and Development of Sociology in Public Health	15
Current Trends in Public Health	18
Growth of Behavioral Science in Public Health	20
Behavioral Science Approaches to Public Health Problems	25
Sociology and Public Health	28
III. The Field of Public Health	32
The Nature of Public Health	32
Development in the United States	34
Organizational Aspects of Public Health	36
Voluntary Health Agencies	38
Private Medicine	40
Changing Needs in Public Health	42
IV. Sociology and Basic Health Processes	47
Ecology and Demography	48
Social Etiology of Disease	53
The Determination and Control of Health Problems	58
Social Responses to Health Problems	64
V. Sociology Applied to Public Health Practice	73
Community Support and Action	78
Individual Participation and Utilization	86
The Epidemiological Model and Health Action	96
VI. Organizational and Occupational Structure of Public Health	100
Structural-Functional Analysis of Public Health Organizations	102
Occupational Analysis of Public Health Field	107

VII.	Activities of Sociologists in Public Health	130
	Research Activities	133
	Teaching Activities	138
	Service Activities	145
	Preparation for Work in Public Health	151
VIII.	Patterns of Collaboration and Interaction	155
	Cultural Differences	159
	Role and Status Problems	160
	Collaboration in an Applied Setting	163
	Resolution of Conflicts	170
IX.	Prospects for the Future	175

FOREWORD

THE PRESENT WORK is the fifth in a series of bulletins on the applications of sociology to various fields of professional practice prepared under the joint sponsorship of the American Sociological Association and Russell Sage Foundation. Previous bulletins have dealt with applications of sociology in the fields of corrections, mental health, education, and military organization.

As Dr. Suchman points out, there is a natural convergence of research interests in public health and sociology that has been evident for some time. This convergence has become much more visible with the mastering of the major contagious diseases and the growing concern with the chronic diseases. When contagious diseases were the major threats to the health of the community, cultural, social-structural, and social-psychological factors, while recognized as certainly present, appeared less strategic than the more specific causal factors as foci of preventive effort. With the rise of the chronic diseases as the major health concerns, the social processes that are the objects of sociological theory and research loom large as strategic elements in control and prevention. What is more, these factors are crucial in the formulation of the programs that must necessarily depend heavily on the intelligent participation by the community whose health needs are to be met.

Dr. Suchman has performed an important service in his clear delineation of the great potential sociology and related disciplines have for sharpening our understanding of the social factors in health and disease, for intelligent planning and mounting of appropriate action programs, and for improving the organizational structure and institutional mechanisms of the health professions themselves.

To this illuminating discussion he has added a perceptive analysis of the problems of cross-disciplinary collaboration between the public health practitioner and the social scientist, together with suggestions for rendering their working relations more effective. Both social scientists and members of the health professions should find the perspective and insight of this work rewarding indeed, emerging as it does out of the experiences of a highly competent social scientist who has devoted over five years to an intensive application of his science to the problems of public health.

In preparing this bulletin, Dr. Suchman has had the benefit of advice from an Advisory Committee consisting of Dr. John A. Clausen, Institute of Human Development at the University of California, Berkeley; Dr. Edward Wellin, Rutgers, The State University; Dr. Benjamin D. Paul, Stanford University School of Medicine; Dr. Richard Williams, National Institute of Mental Health; Dr. Stanley H. King, University Health Services, Harvard University; and Dr. Jack Elinson, School of Public Health and Administrative Medicine, Columbia University.

LEONARD S. COTTRELL, JR.

Russell Sage Foundation
July 1, 1963

ACKNOWLEDGMENTS

As a relative newcomer to the field of public health, the author has been subjected during the past five years to a rather concentrated course of indoctrination—if throwing someone into the water, to sink or swim, can be called indoctrination. However, he has been most fortunate in his choice of life-guards. Collaborating with him on several research projects and on courses in public health were Dr. Jack Elinson of the Columbia University School of Public Health and Administrative Medicine and Dr. George James of the same faculty and the Commissioner of Health of New York City. Both offered freely of their broad knowledge and experience in public health. Dr. James instilled the author with a large measure of his own enthusiasm for a social-psychological approach to modern-day public health problems. The almost daily stream of articles, reprints, news stories "from the desk of Dr. James" were the source of many of the facts and ideas presented in this report.

The author has been encouraged, at all times, in his attempts to apply social science to public health problems by the unfailing support of Dr. Leona Baumgartner, formerly Commissioner of Health of New York City, and Dr. Ray E. Trussell, Executive Officer of the Columbia University School of Public Health and Administrative Medicine, and currently Commissioner of Hospitals for New York City.

The author has had the benefit of a critical reading of his manuscript from his Advisory Committee, composed of Drs. John A. Clausen, Richard H. Williams, Stanley H. King, Edward Wellin, Benjamin D. Paul, and Jack Elinson, and many others who were kind enough to read and comment upon this report in its preliminary version.

To Russell Sage Foundation belongs a large measure of credit for its pioneering efforts at introducing the social sciences into the fields of public health and medicine. Dr. Leonard S. Cottrell, Jr., long a source of personal inspiration, support, and pleasure to the author, provided his usual warm and ready assistance.

Lastly, the author wishes to acknowledge the invaluable help of John H. Marx in collecting materials, in organizing these for presentation, and in critically evaluating the report. The beneficial results of the many hours spent in argument and discussion of the detailed commentaries he prepared may be found on each page of this report.

E. A. S.

I
INTRODUCTION

WHILE THE FIELD OF PUBLIC HEALTH is historically rooted in the social reform movements of the nineteenth century, it is only in recent years that systematic working relationships between social science and public health have become formally established. Current developments in the health field have reawakened the concern of public health workers with social factors in the preventive, therapeutic, and rehabilitative aspects of illness and disease. In turn, the inherently social character of many of the newer public health problems has attracted a rapidly increasing number of sociologists to the field of public health. It is much too early, and changes are occurring much too rapidly, to predict what form this collaboration will finally take; all we can hope to do is to pause for a moment and take a quick look at where we stand and where we are going. But this much is certain—we are entering a period during which public health and the social sciences will be working together to an ever-increasing degree.

The main theme of this bulletin is that a drastic shift in the nature and significance of modern disease patterns and in society's methods for providing medical care has necessitated a change in the focus of public health philosophy and activity. An essential element in this reorientation is the greatly increased need and desirability of collaboration between sociologists and public health practitioners. The large number of congruent or complementary theoretical and methodological approaches shared by the two fields has made the development of working relationships in research, teaching, and service areas mutually profitable. However, the unforeseen rapidity of the growth of such joint efforts, the diffuse, interdisciplinary, multi-faceted nature of social problems in the field of health, and certain inherent characteristics of both fields, one basic and one applied, have created problems and conflicts in this highly functional alliance which have not yet had time to be completely resolved. It is hoped that this bulletin will increase our understanding of the factors underlying some of the major difficulties facing both fields in their efforts to work together and point the way toward more productive collaboration in the future.

The original objective of this bulletin was to point out to sociologists the many opportunities awaiting them in the field of public health. But this now would be like "carrying coals to Newcastle" in view of the large number of sociologists entering the field. In a sense, the market has shifted from seller to buyer, and what may be needed now is a more informed consumer who can make intelligent use of the services of the social scientist. Hence, we have decided to run the risk of writing for two audiences. For the sociologist, we hope to be able to indicate what the *needs* of public health are in relation to the behavioral sciences; while, for the public health professional, we hope to describe the *resources* the behavioral sciences have to offer the field of public health.

In general, we will not attempt to maintain disciplinary purity in our discussion of social concepts and methods applied to public health problems. In our opinion, sociology in public health is basically an applied science. This means that behavioral scientists working in the field must be problem-oriented, not discipline-oriented. Medical sociology will probably develop, in time, its own particular adaptation of social theory and concept in much the same way as other applied fields, such as industrial sociology or educational sociology. Being problem-oriented, a strict and narrow limitation of our presentation to "pure" sociology is not possible. Most public health problems also involve social psychology, anthropology, and, occasionally, economics and political science. The individual, group, or community constituting the target of public health efforts must be seen as an integrated whole, subject to the simultaneous influences of all social, economic, and political forces.

Not only is it important to recognize the interdisciplinary scope of social science in public health; it is also necessary to keep in mind the multi-faceted nature of most social problems in the field of health. Social problems, in general, are interrelated; poverty, housing, fertility, alcoholism, mental disorder, juvenile delinquency, and venereal disease are *not* separate problems; they need to be looked at in combination. The health of the individual and his treatment in illness also represent an intricate complex of biological, physical, social, and cultural forces that need to be taken into account simultaneously. Illness, for example, is rarely an individual problem; almost always it constitutes an important aspect of family maladjustment.

There is one final sense in which sociology applied to public health must avoid disciplinary ethnocentrism. The major accent of an applied social science is upon action; the individual, the group, the community must be induced to do something. But such action in the field of public health cannot be divorced from action in other fields of individual and community welfare. The sociologist working on a community health problem must make use of many different public and voluntary agencies in the health and welfare fields. This will often require a breakdown of professional parochialism and a concerted attack upon a single health problem by many different groups, including public health, private medicine, hospitals, health insurance groups, voluntary health agencies, welfare, public assistance, and social service agencies.

While the main emphasis of this report will be upon the contributions of sociology to public health, it will also be important to point out some of the many ways in which sociology as a science can benefit substantively, theoretically, and methodologically from collaboration with the field of public health. Health, illness, and medical care, *in and of themselves*, constitute significant areas of sociological concern. Until recently, sociology has neglected these important aspects of social life. Health and illness have not been given the same attention as, let us say, education, religion, or industry, while such public health problems as rehabilitation, medical care, population control, and alcoholism have not received the same kind of analysis as other social problem areas, such as divorce, crime, and race relations.

Basic sociological research in the area of public health can serve as a valuable test of existing sociological hypotheses and theories. The subjecting of social theory to the crucial test of prediction and control in real-life situations can provide a most helpful evaluation of the validity of such theory. Concepts such as role and status take on new dimensions when one is forced to examine them in terms of doctor-patient relationships in a treatment situation.

In addition to advancing sociological knowledge, research in the field of public health offers a number of opportunities for methodological progress. The social survey, an important research technique of social science, is also the methodological backbone of epidemiology. In fact, the prospective or longitudinal population survey in public health predates sociological interest in the "panel" or "repeated interview" technique. The growing concern of public health with international health programs offers fertile ground for the development of the comparative or cross-cultural method. Local population laboratories for the study of community health problems can help to advance sociological techniques for the study of community structure and action. The methodology of community public health research is, to a large extent, the methodology of social research.

The development of sociological theory and method within the context of public health research will also provide a more fundamental orientation to current social research on public health problems. Too much of this research remains on the applied or market research level, although some of the most important public health problems demand a much more highly conceptualized approach to interpersonal and intergroup processes. For example, the area of decision-making within the family is critical to such significant public health problems as family participation in public health programs, planned parenthood, and adjustment to chronic illness. Community decision-making processes involving a highly sophisticated analysis of the local power structure and public opinion are basic to the successful introduction of community health programs on fluoridation, radiation, and air pollution. These are highly important public health problems that can be dealt with only by social research utilizing basic social theory.

In general, this bulletin will address itself to the following six questions:

1. What are the current needs in public health that sociology is attempting to meet, and how did these develop?
2. What is the nature of the relationship of sociology to public health? What forces lead to convergence or divergence of the two fields?
3. What contribution does sociology have to make to public health in the understanding and control of health problems?
4. What contribution does sociology have to make to public health in the study and organization of public health structures and personnel?
5. What activities do sociologists in public health engage in; where, how, and with what results?
6. What problems of collaboration exist between sociologists and public health workers, and how are these being met?

In discussing these six questions, we have classified our materials according to their major focus upon the disease process (Chapter IV), the public (Chapter V), or the profession (Chapter VI). This classification of public health into three major areas is somewhat similar to other classifications offered by sociologists studying medical and public health problems. Briefly, we may compare the relationship of the person to the profession with Henderson's analysis of the medical field as a social system involving the interaction of the health actor—medical or professional, and the client—individual or community.[1] The significance of this division lies in its approach to health problems in terms of the interpersonal role relationships between practitioners and recipients. Employing a more problem-oriented approach, Kendall and Merton classify the field of social research in health into four categories: (a) etiology and ecology; (b) variations in response to illness and maintenance of health; (c) organization of health facilities; and (d) professional education and training.[2] In our presentation we have separated etiology from ecology and we view the variations in response to illness apart from the more applied problems of changing such behavior through public health programs.

Wellin comes closest to our own classification by talking about (a) disease (or social pathology with health implications);

(b) behavior and belief (responses to illness and to health programs); and (c) means, agencies, personnel (institutional patterns for management of illness).[3] The most comprehensive classification, and an excellent bibliographical review, is offered by Polgar, who, adopting essentially an anthropological approach, talks about (a) the dynamics of health status; (b) popular health cultures; (c) health personnel; and (d) health action programs. This classification is particularly appropriate to our problem in its focus upon methods of changing health behavior in terms of the characteristics of the disease conditions themselves, the beliefs and behavior of the individuals, and the actions of the public health professionals.[4] Again we note the basic emphasis upon the triad of disease, individual, and profession. The following chapters will focus upon each one of these three in turn.

NOTES TO CHAPTER I

1. Henderson, Lawrence J., "Physician and Patient as a Socia System," *New England Journal of Medicine*, vol. 212, May 2, 1935, pp. 819-823.
2. Kendall, Patricia L., and Robert K. Merton, "Medical Education as a Social Process" in Jaco, E. Gartly, editor, *Patients, Physicians and Illness*. The Free Press, Glencoe, Ill., 1958, pp. 321-350.
3. Wellin, Edward, "Socio-Cultural Factors in Public Health: A Discussion," *Annals of the New York Academy of Sciences*, vol. 84, art. 17, December 8, 1960, p. 1044.
4. Polgar, Steven, "Health and Human Behavior: Areas of Interest Common to the Social and Medical Sciences," *Current Anthropology*, vol. 3, April, 1962, pp. 159-205.

II

THE GROWTH AND DEVELOPMENT OF SOCIOLOGY IN PUBLIC HEALTH

HISTORICALLY, the relationship between the health of the public and social factors is a long and natural one dating back to antiquity.[1] Communities have always been concerned with social conditions that were perceived as threats to the health of their members. The efforts of society to improve and maintain its health may be seen in the prayers and rituals of primitive tribes against pestilence. Evidence of a concern with socioenvironmental factors in health may be found in the ancient civilizations of Egypt, India, and China. Many of the early philosophers and precursors of modern medicine concerned themselves as much with social conditions related to health as with biological factors.

On a broad level, of course, social and cultural factors have always played an important part in determining the way in which public health and medical services were organized. The value system of a society helps to shape the public's attitudes, beliefs, and behavior in regard to health and illness. Health institutions, like all social institutions, reflect a society's definition of what constitutes an acceptable and appropriate organization of health activity. The roles assigned to both the practitioner and the recipient of medical care represent, in large measure, socially prescribed behavior. As an inherently social and cultural activity, public health is thus an integral part of the social system, and can be fully understood only in terms of existing social forces.

Not only has society influenced the health of its members, it has, in turn, been influenced by its public's health. Pestilence and plague have had dramatic effects upon the course of history. As Zinsser points out, typhus fever was largely responsible for

Charles V becoming ruler of the Holy Roman Empire.[2] The decline of early European civilization may be traced to the advent of the malaria mosquito in Greece in 400 B.C. Yellow fever defeated France's attempt to build the Panama Canal, while the tsetse fly helped to shape the political division of southern Africa in the late nineteenth century. To a large extent, the prosperity and security of modern nations continue to depend upon the health and physical well-being of their citizens.

The modern public health movement is a relatively new development, having assumed its present official form only toward the end of the nineteenth century. Part and parcel of the social revolution that accompanied the rise of modern industrial society, it had its origin in the social reform movements of the past century, movements that also included public education and welfare. The organization of the first official public health agency was almost a direct consequence of a social survey by Edwin Chadwick, an *Inquiry into the Sanitary Condition of the Labouring Population of Great Britain*. In this country Lemuel Shattuck's *Report to the Massachusetts Sanitary Commission* was similarly a pioneering effort in both public health and social science. Then followed an era of rapid growth in the administrative organization of public health services and the development of a separate occupation of public health workers. Today each country of the civilized world has developed its own brand of public health organization, strongly reflecting the social and political philosophy of that country. Perhaps the next step in society's efforts to control the way in which the community meets its problems of health and disease is represented by the current rapid development of governmental systems of "socialized" medicine.

The public health movement numbered a great many "giants" during its early pioneering days. Full of the fire of social reform, such men as John Howard, Edwin Chadwick, C.-E. A. Winslow, and Lemuel Shattuck sparked the drive toward better health conditions for the public. As in many social movements, these pioneers were followed by the discoverers and research workers who helped to supply the factual knowledge upon which the movement could progress. These were the great heroes of epidemiology, men like Snow, Goldberger, and Frost, who fought the battles against the plagues and epidemics of the past, who initiated the crusades against cholera, pellagra, and smallpox.

Today, as the public health movement has attained formal status and respectability, these early leaders have given way to the statesmen, administrators, and technicians who labor to translate the ever-increasing knowledge of medical research into daily operating programs for the improved health and well-being of the public. Dwork divides the present administrative leadership of public health into three main categories—the *philosophers* or scholars who blend the behavioral sciences and medicine and who recognize and meet changing trends, the *strategists* or researchers who examine and test ideas, and the *tacticians* who bridge the gulf between ideas and action.[3] Whether or not the public health movement has reached that final stage of development represented by a bureaucracy with a vested interest in securing its own power and in keeping things as they are is a point of great debate today. Certainly, it is one of the dangers of the future.[4]

The growth of public health is also closely linked to the disease patterns of different historical periods and the success with which medical science was able to cope with these threats to the community. In an excellent analysis of the concept of preventive medicine, Anderson and Rosen[5] delineate five patterns of disease over the past one thousand years: (1) leprosy and plague, (2) louse-borne disease and syphilis, (3) gastro-intestinal diseases, (4) tuberculosis and the communicable diseases of childhood, (5) cardiovascular-renal diseases, malignant neoplasms, and accidents. They conclude this list by predicting a sixth pattern, the psychosomatic diseases, characterized by the emergence of social and psychological factors as major forces in health, illness, and medical care.

Paralleling these changing patterns of disease, Alan Gregg divides public health history into three major eras: (1) the era of authority—from antiquity to the beginnings of medical science; (2) the era of research, experimentation, and treatment of specific diseases; and (3) the era of ecology—the modern era, now just beginning, in which the whole patient and the community, rather than the disease entity, become the focus of medical attention.[6] Many of the current problems in public health and medical care spring from the difficulties of this period of transition.

For tomorrow, public health has set itself a further ideal, proclaimed by the World Health Organization in its declaration of the goal of public health as "a state of complete physical, mental and social well-being and not merely the absence of disease or infirmity." This is admittedly an ideal, which like any statement of a creed would be difficult to define in exact terms, but it does set the standard for the basic philosophy of the modern public health movement.

Thus we see that the history and philosophy of public health is an inherent part of the growth of civilization. This history has had its periods of enlightenment and darkness, of humanity and inhumanity; and its prevailing norms and values reflect both this historical background and current social, economic, political, and medical forces. With its roots in medical science, public health is dedicated to the use of the scientific approach both for the discovery of new knowledge and for the evaluation of existing programs. It believes that research is basic to progress and it constantly seeks to advance the frontiers of new knowledge by means of medical, epidemiological, and, more recently, behavioral science research. As a field of action, it is imbued with a strong sense of public service and is highly aware of its professional and moral responsibility to improve the health of the public. It approaches this task with a value system that presupposes the ability of man to control himself and his environment and, through planning, to attain a state of better physical and mental well-being.

Current Trends in Public Health

During the bacteriological era, public health had little need for the behavioral sciences. Under the impetus of communicable disease control programs, it was hard at work establishing its legitimacy as a public service and defining its sphere of activity. Vast new discoveries in medical science concerning the communicable diseases—discoveries that could be administered in a routine fashion by an organized public health service—provided both the opportunity and means for acceptance and growth. There was a tremendous job to be done and there was little time or need for a concern with behavioral forces.

These early efforts were highly successful in the western world and the communicable diseases began to disappear[7]—only to be replaced by a new type of disease that did not respond to immunization or control of sanitary conditions. These so-called diseases of civilization—the chronic, degenerative diseases such as cancer, heart disease, arthritis, diabetes, and mental disorders—rapidly rose to the top of the morbidity and mortality tables until today we find the major public health programs striving desperately but rather unsuccessfully to control them.

These chronic diseases created a whole new set of problems for the field of public health—problems relating to both their prevention and care, if not cure. At the heart of many of these problems was the nature of the relationship of organized health services to the public. People now had to be persuaded, rather than compelled, to take advantage of preventive measures. The chronically ill did not present the same kind of apparent threat to the public's health as individuals with an infectious, communicable disease. The formal authority and legal sanctions so crucial in the fight against communicable disease were displaced by appeals for community support and by inducements to individuals to take advantage of public health programs and facilities. The health of the individual became largely a personal rather than a public matter.

Furthermore, the dividing line between preventive and therapeutic medicine was becoming increasingly difficult to draw. The chronic diseases could not be prevented in the traditional sense of halting the development of the disease entirely. Some of them could be detected in their early stages but, even so, they could rarely be cured, only slowed down or prevented from developing further. Therapy, in this sense, was largely preventive and rehabilitative, not curative. Drugs were of less avail than the motivation and ability of the individual to change his customary behavior and way of life. These chronic diseases were long-term illnesses during which problems of adjustment and rehabilitation loomed large. Occurring as they did most frequently among older people, many of whom could not bear the high costs of such long-term care, medical welfare became an increasingly difficult challenge to public health.

With these changes came the need for developing new relationships between public health and the public, on one hand, and public health and organized private medicine on the other. The old established public health programs based on authority were replaced by new voluntary programs requiring community support and individual motivation. The division of labor with private medicine, always a source of some contention, became one of open conflict over the provision of medical care for the chronically ill—especially the indigent and the old. Public health now entered an era of new competition—a competition with other community interests opposed to certain health measures that could no longer be justified by the threat of epidemics; with business interests that had found the health field financially profitable, such as drugs and vitamins; with other powerful economic interests engaged in activities deemed harmful to the public's health, such as the tobacco, food additive, and insecticide industries; with private medicine over the quantity, and perhaps even more important, the quality of medical care for the public. And as public health assumed a less dramatic role than preventing major epidemics, it had to take its place alongside other needed public services, such as urban redevelopment and education, in competition for the increasingly scarce tax dollar.

Thus we find the field of public health today intimately and bewilderingly involved with such "nonmedical" problems as organizing political support for fluoridation, seeking legislation to provide adequate medical care, securing community support for voluntary health measures, motivating individuals to take advantage of mass screening programs or to change their eating, drinking, and living habits. This is the current state of need out of which public health is now turning to the behavioral sciences.

Growth of Behavioral Science in Public Health

In an excellent description of the role of social forces in the development of medical care, Roemer and Elling date the modern origins of "medical sociology" to the sixteenth century, during which the major epidemic diseases such as plague and typhus fever were traced to contagiousness (a social process), diseases of miners to their occupational status, and scurvy to eating habits.[8] In the seventeenth century such men as Petty and Gaunt developed mortality tables related to social group characteristics. The eighteenth century was called a "period of enlightenment," during which sweeping proposals were put forth for better safeguarding of the health of the working classes. Early attempts during the nineteenth century to develop social health legislation were sidetracked by the great discoveries in bacteriology, which provided such immediate practical rewards that it is little wonder that the energies of public health research and action were almost completely devoted to the conquest of the communicable diseases. It remained for the twentieth century once again to revive the movement toward broad social studies and social action aimed at the organization of public health and medical care.

In regard to current developments, Roemer and Elling place particular emphasis upon social and political efforts to introduce public systems of health insurance. In the early twentieth century such men as Sydenstricker,[9] Davis,[10] and Moore[11] analyzed the relationship of health needs to health resources in the United States, largely in terms of "medical economics." The most significant and influential work of this period was the 28-volume report of the Committee on the Costs of Medical Care completed during the depression of 1932.[12] These various studies raised serious questions concerning the adequacy of medical organization in the United States and pointed the way toward the growth of governmental interest in the provision of medical care.

Among sociologists, Bernhard J. Stern was one of the first to show an interest in health problems. His monograph, *Social Factors in Medical Progress*, offered a historical analysis of resistances to medical innovation.[13] Lynd, in his study of Middletown, included a chapter on problems of health. However, for the most part, sociologists did not evince an early interest in social problems related to health. This was left mainly to the economists who in the 1920's and 1930's became concerned with problems in the provision of medical care. The debate over the proper financing of the public's health still remains at the forefront of the current sociopolitical scene.

The fact that public health is today turning to the behavioral sciences represents a need that has largely been forced upon the field by changes both in the patterns of disease and in the social organization of medical care. Many of the current problems of social epidemiology in relation to the chronic degenerative diseases necessitate a sociocultural approach. The consequences of illness, especially as they create problems of long-term care and rehabilitation, directly involve social factors. Participation in mass screening programs, the utilization of existing health facilities, and community support for public health measures are only some of the problems facing public health today that require a knowledge of social action. The organization of health services, including the establishment of health insurance plans for medical care, present very real challenges in social economics. Such current social problems as overpopulation, old age, alcoholism, narcotics addiction, juvenile delinquency, housing, and so on are intrinsically bound up with public health concerns. It is little wonder that in 1953 the American Public Health Association unanimously passed this resolution: "That the American Public Health Association encourage collaboration between public health workers and social scientists to better promote the utilization of social science findings toward the solution of public health problems."

The need is there, and patterns of interaction are slowly being established but, to a large extent, the atmosphere is still a mixture of resistance and welcome. Some of the causes of this resistance have been pointed out by Dr. Hugh Leavell.

> Social science research takes time and is expensive, and findings are not easily demonstrable to those unfamiliar with the technical language and methods. Results of research are apt to carry obvious implications for social change, naturally resisted by vested interests. The multi-disciplinary teamwork urgently needed for many investigations is difficult to bring about successfully. There are some divisions among the ranks of the social scientists themselves, and the field needs a more unified approach and a broad theoretical concept upon which further research may be based.[14]

Other reasons for the reluctance of public health workers to embrace the social sciences include the lack of any clear-cut directions about how social science can be used in concrete service programs and the uneasiness of the public health worker in the face of abstract, complex social concepts and inconclusive, often nonrigorous, research findings. In addition, the social factors in public health force the health worker to enter the political arena of social policy-making—an arena that is both strange and threatening.

On the whole, however, the reception that public health has given to the behavioral sciences has been enthusiastic—at times a little too enthusiastic. In some instances, there has been a naive overestimation of what the behavioral sciences had to contribute, resulting in a somewhat too uncritical acceptance of behavioral science concepts and personnel. To some extent, behavioral scientists have even become status symbols in the field of public health—signs of progressive thinking.

We have only to look at some basic facts and figures to comprehend the tremendous spurt in activity on the part of sociologists in the field of public health during the past fifteen years. When the American Sociological Association set up sections on specific aspects of sociology in 1959, one of the first to receive the prescribed 200 members was the Section on Medical Sociology. Within the first year of its existence, the membership had climbed past the 500 mark, to reach 878 members in 1962, the Association's largest section. A comparison of the changes in the major fields of competence among members of the American Sociological Association between 1950 and 1959 showed medical sociology at the head of the list, with the highest percentage gain (723 per cent, or an absolute increase from 26 to 188 members).[15]

An analysis by Simpson of the various fields of activity within sociology listed medical sociology as one of the three general fields out of 23 that showed an increase in the number of Ph.D.'s in the period 1950 to 1959. Medical sociology was also one of the four fields with a steadily increasing proportion of papers presented at the annual meetings of the American Sociological Association, from 3.8 per cent in the 1946 to 1949 period to 13.4 per cent in the 1955 to 1959 period. This growth was also evident in the proportion of articles published in the *American Sociological Review*, from 2.7 per cent during 1946 to 1949 to 7.7 per cent during 1955 to 1959. Significantly, and perhaps indicative of an "academic lag," an analysis of undergraduate college courses given in sociology finds medical sociology poorly represented.[16] This is probably due to the newness of the field, the currently strong emphasis upon "applied" research, and the absence of any well-integrated body of knowledge to be communicated to the student.

In 1957 the Health Information Foundation conducted a survey of 216 behavioral scientists known to be engaged in research in the health field full time or part time. While the representativeness of this sample is unknown, overwhelmingly the major field of study mentioned by the individuals surveyed was sociology, 79 per cent, with psychology and anthropology sharing second place with 9 per cent each.[17] Each year the Health Information Foundation makes an inventory of social and economic research in health. This inventory is based upon questionnaires mailed to organizations and individuals concerned with studies of health levels; of health resources-services, facilities, personnel; and of behavioral and economic aspects of health. The 1960 edition of this inventory listed 1,035 projects, of which 452 were new projects. Each new edition has seen a marked increase in the number of projects listed, and this increase may be expected to continue.

Under grants from Russell Sage Foundation, social science programs have been established within the New York City, Philadelphia, and Puerto Rico Departments of Health. Russell Sage Foundation has also been highly instrumental in the organization of social science programs in the Schools of Public Health at Harvard University and the University of California, in Berkeley. While these activities represent pioneering efforts, there can be little doubt that they will be followed by more and more such programs, especially in view of the Social Science Training Grants program of the National Institute of Mental Health.

Sociologists may increasingly be found in schools of public health and in operating health agencies. Almost all of the graduate schools of public health have one or more sociologists as members. Many of the voluntary and public health agencies now employ sociologists in their research and service programs. These range from the United States Public Health Service on a national level through the state health departments, to the local city and county health departments. Similarly, many of the voluntary health agencies, such as the American Heart Association and the National Foundation, have turned to sociologists for consultation about their research and service programs.

These are only some of the current activities relating to sociology and the field of public health. This list could easily be expanded by many more references to individual programs, conferences, and so on. Six journals have devoted special issues to articles dealing with the social, psychological, and anthropological aspects of health—*Journal of Social Issues* (1952), *Social Problems* (1956), *Health Education Journal* (1957), *Human Organization* (1958), *Journal of Health and Human Behavior* (1962), and the *Annals of the American Academy of Political and Social Science* (1963). Finally, certain inevitable signs of growing pains have also made their appearance—a rather elementary textbook devoted to medical sociology,[18] a much more comprehensive and thoughtful analysis of the doctor-patient relationship for use in the medical curriculum,[19] two readers containing collections of articles in the field,[20,21] a new journal,[22] a handbook of medical sociology,[23] and the present bulletin.

Behavioral Science Approaches to Public Health Problems

At the present stage of development, there is little agreement concerning the differentiations or boundaries among the various social science disciplines as these relate to different aspects of public health and medical care. For the most part, the distinctions that have been made are quite arbitrary and reflect a division of labor rather than any inherent differences in theory or method.

The Behavioral Sciences. In this report we will accept the conventional distinction between the behavioral sciences as referring to those academic disciplines that deal most directly with human behavior—for example, social anthropology, social psychology, and sociology—and the social sciences as indicative of a wider range of interest, including economics and political science. Although our focus will be upon the relationship of sociology to public health, we will feel free to introduce other social sciences, especially social psychology and social anthropology, in our analysis and discussion of public health problems or action. It is difficult, perhaps even unwarranted, to attempt to maintain an academic purity along disciplinary lines when working in an applied field such as public health. The fractionation of man and society that takes place in the university must give way to the whole man or community in real life.

It is our belief that while the current situation prohibits any clear-cut division of either the behavioral science disciplines or the professional fields of health and medical care, it does demand a keen awareness of the kinds of problems created by this "generalist" approach and it does offer a significant challenge to further conceptual analysis. The trend today is toward weakening rather than strengthening the lines of separation between the behavioral science disciplines and the health fields. Thus we tend to speak of the behavioral sciences as dealing with all aspects of human behavior regardless of academic discipline and of social medicine as involving not only the patient but the social group and society to which he belongs. There is little doubt that each social science discipline and health field is partner to the other—and progress will be made in the direction of an increasing integration of disciplinary fields and health services. Future developments will make it more difficult and less profitable to maintain rigid boundary lines or to debate where one aspect of social science or public health ends and another begins.

Health and Medical Care Fields. There is no hard and fast delineation for the field of public health. Public health represents a whole complex of diverse activities calling upon many different academic disciplines and professions. All of these separate parts are drawn together around the common goal of public health—the protection and promotion of the health of the people. Public health lays no serious claims to either distinct theoretical formulations or research methods, although, of course, it has emphasized certain content areas and research techniques as more applicable to its objectives. This is particularly true of epidemiology which, both as subject matter and research method, occupies a central position in the training and activities of public health professionals. As we shall see later, this core of public health "science" is strongly akin to the social science areas of demography and ecology and the social survey research method.

The most general term applied to the place of the social sciences in health is that of "social medicine." In Europe, especially England, this term refers largely to the field of public health and preventive medicine with strong overtones of social action. Halliday states that social medicine "has a very floating meaning at present, being used in Europe as a synonym for state-controlled medicine and in Britain as an alternative to preventive medicine in all its aspects."[24] In the United States the term tends to become confused with "socialized" medicine with all of its political and value overtones and, despite some early attempts to secure its adoption, it is not now widely used. To some extent, the term "medical sociology" has become more acceptable, although this term is probably too narrowly focused on sociological factors to be satisfactory to the other behavioral science disciplines.

In a highly interesting and informative historical analysis of the growth of interaction between the social sciences, medicine, and public health, Rosen links social medicine to policy and action in the health field. Thus, he concludes, "Social medicine is an applied discipline" tied to problems of medical and public health practice. "Medical sociology," on the other hand, has a more basic social science orientation and is concerned with a broader approach to the role of social forces in health and medical care. He suggests a new designation to represent the increased breadth of these social science interests—a "sociology of health."[25]

The present status of medical sociology is reviewed by Freeman, Levine, and Reeder in an analysis which stresses its applied characteristics and, in fact, takes the position that, "There are no reasons for the development of unique or special theories in medical sociology."[26] While it is undoubtedly true that, as a branch of sociology, medical sociology must reflect the theoretical foundations of sociology as a discipline, it is also the case that as of today medical sociology has only made use of existing social theory in a rather haphazard fashion. There are many aspects of social theory with high potential relevance for medical sociology that have not been adequately exploited, especially in the area of social control. A sociologist has yet to produce the kind of integration of theory and subject matter in the health field that, for example, Moore and others have accomplished for the industrial field.[27]

Sociology and Public Health

Since our primary concern is with sociology and public health, we will limit further discussion to an analysis of the theoretical and methodological congruences of these two areas only. It is our contention that sociology and public health have a close affinity in terms of unit of study, theory, and method. They share a common concern with *populations* of individuals, a theoretical orientation toward abstract *generalizations*, and a methodological approach that emphasizes *quantitative*, statistical methods. Sociology and public health also share a problem focus that tends to draw them together. This can be seen historically in the common origins of both fields in the area of social reform. It can be seen today in the increasing overlap between the two fields in relation to such social and health problem areas as population control, old age, juvenile delinquency, and mental retardation.

In regard to the unit of study, both fields are largely concerned with the behavior of groups of individuals rather than single individuals, and have as one of their major objectives the description and explanation of incidence and prevalence rates for whole populations. Demography and ecology are important areas of study for both fields. Each field stresses actuarial or probabilistic prediction for which the behavior of any specific individual in the sample is relatively unimportant. The type of prediction that predominates in any field is crucial for structuring both the conceptual thinking and research activities of that field. Sharing this common emphasis on actuarial prediction creates a highly significant bond between sociology and public health. In regard to applied programs, both social action and public health are also aimed at large numbers of individuals within the community and, for many purposes, it is irrelevant whether any particular individual is reached by any specific program.

Methodologically, the focus of sociology and public health is mainly, again recognizing certain exceptions, upon larger social systems such as institutions, communities, and social classes. Both sociology and public health emphasize the macroscopic (breadth) point of view, which necessarily means a large-scale community approach utilizing mass surveys and field experiments. The concern of sociology and public health with large numbers has resulted in the development in both fields of a quantitative methodology and statistical techniques for the analysis of multiple variables. Social and public health research designs attempt to approximate the experimental model of proof through the use of standardization procedures for controlling extraneous or intervening variables. The epidemiological method and the social survey method have similar sampling, interviewing, instrument design, and analysis problems. As we shall see in a later chapter, each field has developed a somewhat greater sophistication in certain aspects of the population survey and each has something to gain from sharing this methodological knowledge.

Theoretically, public health and sociology focus on social systems and large-scale collectivities that are intrinsically dynamic, open systems. The models used to describe these open systems are primarily rational models in which each of the parts functions to maximize the efficiency of the whole and acts somewhat independently of the whole. Open systems have the advantage of allowing change and thus there is in public health and sociology an implied value assumption that new stimuli can react upon the separate components of the system in order to make one or another of them more rational.

In the rational systems developed by sociology and public health, the various components of the system are relatively independent of each other and are integrated by the criterion of functional efficiency. A stimulus impinging upon one component of a rational system model will not necessarily result in compensation or readjustment by another component of the system, and the various components of the system become evaluated in terms of their contribution to the functional efficiency of the total system.

Thus the common theoretical and methodological foci of the behavioral science discipline of sociology and of the field of public health lead us to conclude that the sociological approach has a "natural" contribution to make to the study of problems in the field of public health.

NOTES TO CHAPTER II

1. An excellent bibliography on the historical background and philosophy of public health, compiled by John J. Hanlon, Fred B. Rogers, and George Rosen, "A Bookshelf of the History and Philosophy of Public Health," appears in the *American Journal of Public Health*, vol. 50, April, 1960, pp. 445–458.
2. Zinsser, Hans, *Rats, Lice and History*. Little, Brown and Co., Boston, 1935.
3. Dwork, Ralph, "Health Administration Viewpoint," *American Journal of Public Health*, vol. 51, July, 1961, pp. 1018–1020.
4. A recent editorial in the *American Journal of Public Health* exhorts the public health officer of today to assert his responsibility for leadership on public health issues. Referring to fluoridation, it states: "Last but not least—on various ceremonial occasions, we express our filial piety for our public health ancestors, but we seemingly forget that we can also learn from them. Lemuel Shattuck, Stephen Smith, Dorman B. Eaton, and the others did not shrink from the political arena when necessary. They were not afraid to stand up and be counted, and they called a spade a spade. Certainly we can do no less today." Editorial, "Fluoridation: The Case for Action," *American Journal of Public Health*, vol. 51, April, 1961, p. 599.
5. Anderson, Odin W., and George Rosen, *An Examination of the Concept of Preventive Medicine*. Health Information Foundation, Research Series 12, New York, 1960, pp. 4–6.
6. Gregg, Alan, "The Future Health Officer's Responsibility: Past, Present and Future," *American Journal of Public Health*, vol. 46, November, 1956, pp. 1384–1389.
7. Communicable diseases still constitute a major threat in the underdeveloped areas of the world, and international public health still has an enormous job ahead—a task which has been characterized as one of substituting the chronic for the communicable diseases as the main causes of death.
8. Roemer, Milton I., and Ray H. Elling, "Sociological Research on Medical Care," *Journal of Health and Human Behavior*, vol. 4, Spring, 1963, pp. 49–68. An extensive bibliography of almost 100 pages on past and present publications in the field of sociology and public health, compiled by Ozzie G. Simmons, "Social Research in Health and Medicine: A Bibliography" is presented in Freeman, Howard, Sol Levine, and Leo G. Reeder, editors, *Handbook of Medical Sociology*, Prentice-Hall, Inc., Englewood Cliffs, N. J., 1963, pp. 493–581.
9. Sydenstricker, Edgar, *Health and Environment*. McGraw-Hill Book Co., New York, 1933.
10. Davis, Michael M., *Clinics, Hospitals and Health Centers*. Harper and Bros., New York, 1927. See also *Medical Care for Tomorrow*, Harper and Bros., New York, 1955.
11. Moore, Harry H., *American Medicine and the People's Health*. D. Appleton and Co., New York, 1927.

THE GROWTH AND DEVELOPMENT OF SOCIOLOGY 31

12. Falk, J. S., C. R. Rorem, and M. D. Ring, *The Costs of Medical Care.* Committee on the Costs of Medical Care, Publication No. 27 (summary volume). University of Chicago Press, Chicago, 1933.
13. Stern, Bernhard J., *Social Factors in Medical Progress.* Columbia University Press, New York, 1927.
14. Leavell, Hugh R., "Medical Progress: Contributions of the Social Sciences to the Solution of Health Problems," *New England Journal of Medicine,* vol. 247, December 4, 1952, p. 894.
15. Riley, Mathilda White, "Membership of the American Sociological Association, 1950–59," *American Sociological Review,* vol. 26, December, 1961, p. 925.
16. Simpson, Richard L., "Expanding and Declining Fields in American Sociology," *American Sociological Review,* vol. 26, June, 1961, pp. 458–466.
17. Anderson, Odin W., and Milvoy S. Seacat, *The Behavioral Scientists and Research in the Health Field.* Health Information Foundation, Research Series 1, New York, 1957.
18. Hawkins, Norman G., *Medical Sociology.* Charles C Thomas, Springfield, Ill., 1958. It is interesting to note a much earlier book with this title, *Medical Sociology,* by James P. Warbasse, D. Appleton and Co., New York, 1909, which contained a collection of essays on the relation between medicine and sociology.
19. Bloom, Samuel W., *The Doctor and His Patient.* Russell Sage Foundation, New York, 1963.
20. Jaco, E. Gartly, editor, *Patients, Physicians and Illness.* The Free Press, Glencoe, Ill., 1958.
21. Apple, Dorrian, editor, *Sociological Studies of Health and Sickness.* McGraw-Hill Book Co., New York, 1960.
22. *Journal of Health and Human Behavior,* the first issue of which appeared in Fall, 1960.
23. Freeman, Howard, Sol Levine, and Leo G. Reeder, editors, *Handbook of Medical Sociology.* Prentice-Hall, Inc., Englewood Cliffs, N. J., 1963.
24. Halliday, J. L., *Psychosocial Medicine:* A Study of the Sick Society. William W. Norton and Co., New York, 1948.
25. Rosen, George, "The Evolution of Social Medicine" in Freeman, Levine, and Reeder, editors, *op. cit.,* pp. 50–51. This article also offers a comprehensive history of the development of social medicine.
26. Freeman, Howard, Sol Levine, and Leo G. Reeder, "Present Status of Medical Sociology" in Freeman, Levine, and Reeder, editors, *op. cit.,* pp. 475–476. For an earlier summary of the status of medical sociology, see Freeman, Howard, and Leo G. Reeder, "Medical Sociology: A Review of the Literature," *American Sociological Review,* vol. 22, February, 1957, pp. 74–81.
27. Moore, Wilbert E., *Industrial Relations and the Social Order.* Macmillan Co., New York, 1947.

III

THE FIELD OF PUBLIC HEALTH

A SOCIOLOGIST contemplating work in the field of public health should know something about its history and traditions, its current status, and its outlook for the future. This orientation will be helpful both to those sociologists who wish to study public health as a significant aspect of the modern social system and to those who are more interested in applying their sociological knowledge to the solution of problems in an important area of social welfare. Too often social scientists enter an applied field without adequate knowledge of the history and philosophy, goals and organization of that field, only to find themselves committing numerous professional and interpersonal blunders. Of necessity, we will not be able to give full recognition to the wide range and rapidly changing nature of public health work. Furthermore, this summary of the field of public health will be highly selective, emphasizing those aspects of particular relevance and interest to sociologists.[1]

The Nature of Public Health

Public health, at various stages in its history, has been defined as environmental sanitation, preventive medical science, and most recently, as the promotion of positive health or the attainment of the highest level of physical, mental, and social well-being. Most current definitions place particular stress upon three factors: (1) the prevention or control of disease, (2) through organized community efforts, (3) aimed at special groups of persons. In recent years, because of changes in both the social system and medical practice, these three aspects have taken on new meanings which make it increasingly difficult to separate the public from the private sectors of health.

First, organized community efforts have greatly expanded in almost all areas of health and medical care. Both official and voluntary health agencies have increased their services to the public and have assumed a greater initiative in making public health decisions. Perhaps nowhere is this more apparent than in the provision of medical care. In the face of rising medical costs, the community, led largely by organized labor, has demanded and is receiving a stronger voice in determining how medical care is to be distributed and paid for. It appears inevitable that the community of the future will provide a higher proportion of the necessary medical services.

Secondly, the concept of special groups of people, usually implying the medically indigent, is rapidly being expanded to include entire subgroups of the population, such as elderly people, infants, and young children. In addition, such major segments of the population as the physically handicapped and mentally retarded are increasingly falling within the scope of public health responsibility.

Finally, the definition of prevention, especially in relation to the chronic degenerative diseases, now includes communitywide mass screening programs and preventive measures that relate to the individual's continuing way of life and not just to single immunizations or acts. Tertiary prevention, or rehabilitation, further expands the territory of public health to cover many cases requiring long-term care. Thus public health today is vitally concerned with a wide range of problems that go far beyond the traditional limits of community programs in environmental sanitation and the prevention of epidemics.

Seven of the major elements underlying the practice of public health are listed by Roney as follows: "(1) The prevention of avoidable significant illness or disability or premature death; (2) in any stage of the range of the condition—the disease spectrum; (3) in a community; (4) by control of causative agent, human and environmental factors; (5) through activities of public health technicians; (6) utilizing public funds; (7) with the support and cooperation of interested community groups and individuals, and the acquiescence and understanding of the majority of the community."[2]

From this description it is clear that public health is a combination of art and science. It represents the application of medical knowledge derived from the medical sciences to the problems of community and individual health through the use of sociological and psychological knowledge derived from the behavioral sciences. Almost all current descriptions of public health work stress the importance of a knowledge of human behavior for the effective conduct of public health programs. Some public health people have gone so far as to characterize public health as fundamentally a social science which is only technically related to the field of medicine.[3]

Development in the United States[4]

The growth of organized public health in the United States dates back to the middle of the nineteenth century. New York City in 1866 is credited with having established the first metropolitan Board of Health. In 1872 the American Public Health Association was formed. In 1879, following an epidemic of yellow fever, a National Board of Health was formed, but this lasted only four years. The United States Public Health Service, the most important present-day federal health agency, came into existence in 1912 as a continuation of the Public Health and Marine Hospital Service, organized in 1902. It, in turn, was a continuation of the Marine Hospital Service, which was authorized by Congress in 1798.

The year 1912 marks the beginning of the rapid and steady growth of the public health movement in the United States. It lead to the Social Security Act of 1935, which was enacted "for the purpose of assisting states, counties, health districts, and other political subdivisions of the states in establishing and maintaining adequate public health service, including the training of personnel for state and local health work. . . ."

The activities of the United States Public Health Service were broadened in 1937 with the creation of the first of the national institutes of health, the National Cancer Institute, which was to set the pattern for a number of such institutes in the next decade. Under President Franklin D. Roosevelt's major program of reorganization, a Federal Security Agency was created in 1939, to be followed by two further reorganizations in 1944 and 1954. Other significant developments of this period included the Hill-

Burton Act for hospital construction (1946) and the National Mental Health Act (1946). The next four years witnessed the formation of four other national health institutes: the National Heart Institute (1948), the National Institute of Mental Health (1949), the National Institute of Neurological Diseases and Blindness (1950), and the National Institute of Arthritis and Metabolic Diseases (1950). The latest institute, authorized in 1962, has special relevance for the behavioral sciences, a National Institute of Child Health and Human Development for work in the area of "normal and abnormal development of the human being."

The future mission and organizational structure of the Public Health Service has been the subject of a recent detailed analysis by a Study Group on the Mission and Organization of the Public Health Service.[5] The purpose of this study was to review the structure and function of the Public Health Service in the face of a rapidly changing picture of health needs and resources. The present decade, 1960 to 1970, was seen as "a time for decision in fields related to American health." Two broad areas were expected to require the greatest attention in the next decade: the physical environment (the development and application of new, more efficient techniques to measure, evaluate, and control natural and artificial factors in the environment that affect health and safety) and comprehensive health care (the development of adequate supplies of well-qualified personnel, appropriate facilities, new and more efficient methods to render comprehensive services to the American people). Of particular interest to behavioral scientists was the recommendation by this Study Group to establish a single division which would be "a major focus for studies in the social and behavioral sciences," including community mental health services, alcoholism, juvenile delinquency, and drug addiction.

Paralleling this rapid development of the national health service, we find a concurrent increase in local and state health departments, in voluntary health agencies, and in professional schools of public health. Although in existence only since World War I, these schools now occupy an established place in the field of public health education. There are currently 12 graduate schools of public health that give either the degree of Doctor of Public Health or Master of Public Health.[6] Several of these schools of public health have recently instituted social science programs.

The continuation of this rapid growth in public health activities is inevitable; in fact, there is some reason to believe that we are now entering an era in which the fight against illness and disease and the organization of medical care facilities will become areas of major social and political concern.

Organizational Aspects of Public Health[7]

Public health activities may be divided into service, training, and research, although there is a great deal of overlap among these activities in any single organization. The service or operational aspects of public health are by far the most significant, since public health is that branch of government charged with the protection of the health of the community on a day-to-day basis. As of 1960, there were more than 1,500 local health units in the United States, as well as various state and federal health services. It is estimated that close to 95 per cent of the United States population is serviced by local health units, although many of these may be quite inadequate according to modern standards.[8]

The major responsibilities of these health units include the operation of service programs, such as a communicable disease control, the provision of public health nursing services, the regulation or control of sanitary conditions in public establishments, laboratory services, the operation of child health stations and school health services, the education of the public regarding health habits, and the collection and analysis of vital statistics. The scope of these activities, of course, varies tremendously from the small county health department where the staff might consist of a health officer, a public health engineer, and a public health nurse to a large city health department such as New York's, consisting of more than 5,000 employees.

An excellent listing of public health activities on a community level may be obtained from the *Community Guide to an Evaluation of Health Programs*, prepared by the American Public Health Association, to serve as an instrument for evaluating both public and voluntary health programs.[9] This guide presents detailed indices for 16 phases of public health work: (1) personnel, facilities, and services, (2) public health problems, (3) community health education and staff training, (4) communicable disease control, (5) tuberculosis control, (6) venereal disease control, (7) maternal health, (8) infant and preschool health, (9) school health, (10) adult health, (11) accident prevention, (12) water supplies and excreta disposal, (13) food control, (14) milk control, (15) housing, and (16) financial support for local health work. These topic headings cover most of the current programs carried on by public health agencies.

In addition to the local health units, each state has a separate department responsible for public health. For the most part, the state departments do not provide direct personal services, but concentrate on helping local health units.[10] On the federal level, we find a great complexity of agencies concerned with public health. Mountin and Flook in their *Guide to Health Organization in the United States* list more than 50 federal agencies engaged in health work.[11] This pamphlet provides a good summary of the organization of all health services in the United States.

The United States Public Health Service is, of course, the principal federal agency concerned with public health. This organization operates a wide range of research and service programs, as well as being responsible for financial grants to nonfederal agencies for research and service. A separate agency, the Children's Bureau, is responsible for health services to mothers and children. Other programs of interest to public health are to be found in the Department of Agriculture, the Department of the Interior, and the Food and Drug Administration.

Finally, it is important to mention the increasing number of public health activities on the international level. The United States has taken an active part in the promotion of world health, largely through the International Health Division of the Public Health Service and the Agency for International Development of the Department of State. These units are concerned with special health missions to foreign countries, with programs on the international exchange of health personnel, with international agreements on sanitary conventions and regulations, with representation at international health conferences, and so forth. The Agency for International Development works with foreign countries throughout the world, especially in the provision of technical assistance in public health matters. This organization also awards fellowships for advanced training in the United States and elsewhere to public health workers.

The World Health Organization, an agency of the United Nations, has taken the lead in international health with its recognition that "the health of all peoples is fundamental to the attainment of peace and security." The function of WHO is to direct and coordinate international health work, to provide various technical services, such as epidemiology and vital statistics, and to help countries strengthen and improve their health services. The following six problems have been given major attention by WHO: malaria, maternal and child health, venereal disease, environmental sanitation, and nutrition. The work of these international health programs provides a great many opportunities for sociologists interested in public health on the international or cross-cultural level.

Voluntary Health Agencies

The picture of public health organization in the United States would not be complete without a brief mention of the relationships between public health, voluntary health agencies, and private medicine. In order to understand the system of medical care in the United States today, one must be sensitive to the various conflicting forces in the field of health. This subject is a highly controversial one and involves basic values and assumptions concerning the role of government in providing for the health of its citizens. We cannot go into the details of this conflict, but suffice it to say that as of the present there is a great deal of room for improvement in the cooperative relationships between public health, private medicine, and voluntary health agencies.

Looking first at the voluntary health agencies, we are struck with their number and variety. Since World War II more than 100,000 national, regional, and local voluntary health and welfare agencies have come into being, with a total solicitation from the public of about one and a half billion dollars annually. Hanlon divides these into the following five categories: first, and most important, is a large group of agencies supported by citizen contributions and donations. They are subdivided into those that are concerned with specific diseases, such as the American Cancer Society and the National Tuberculosis Association; those concerned with certain organs or structures of the body, such as the National Society for the Prevention of Blindness and the National Society for Crippled Children; those concerned with the health and welfare of special groups, such as the Maternity Center Association; and those concerned with certain phases of health and welfare, such as the National Safety Council. The second large group of voluntary agencies consists of foundations financed by private funds. Prominent among these are the Rockefeller Foundation, Kellogg Foundation, Commonwealth Fund, Milbank Memorial Fund, and Markle Foundation. The third group of voluntary health agencies is made up of professional associations, such as the American Public Health Association, American Medical Association, National League for Nursing, and the like. The fourth group would consist of such integrating agencies as health councils and community chests, foremost among which are the National Health Council and the United Community Chest. There are now more than a thousand of these multiple interest groups on the local, state, and national levels. A fifth group of nonofficial agencies would comprise those commercial organizations that are interested in promoting public health: large insurance companies and industries concerned with the manufacture and sale of such products as soap, sugar, milk, and meat.[12]

A study of voluntary agencies by Gunn and Platt lists eight basic functions of these organizations: pioneering, demonstration, education, supplementation of official activities, the guarding of citizen interest in health, promotion of health legislation, group planning and coordination, and the development of well-rounded community health programs.[13] To these we might add the support of research, an activity that has become increasingly popular with these agencies, perhaps largely because of its strong public appeal.

MacIntosh stresses a kind of dynamism that is largely lacking from present-day voluntary health agencies, which seem to be more concerned with perpetuating their existence than eliminating the health problems, and hence themselves. According to MacIntosh, such voluntary organizations should always be on "the spreading edge of a movement," "should have enough faith to take risks," and should aim at "self-extinction."[14]

A recent evaluation of voluntary health agencies by Hamlin concluded that these organizations were not functioning as well as they should. He found that "the proliferation of agencies and the expansion of their activities have not always paralleled the public need or interest. Furthermore, the machinery of many voluntary agencies has become antiquated, patched up, and at times jealously self-centered."[15] The Hamlin study recommended that national health organizations be placed under government regulation and be required to establish standardized accounting systems. This study also proposed that the number of local affiliates be drastically reduced.

Private Medicine

Underlying the conflict between public health and private medicine is the age-old controversy of governmental versus private provision of medical care. The growth of a social welfare philosophy in the United States, combined with a die-hard determination of organized medicine to keep medical care on a "fee-for-service" free enterprise basis, has established the battlefield upon which the future of medical care in the United States will be shaped. The case for public health has been made in a statement of the Joint Committee on Medical Care of the American Public Health Association and the American Public Welfare Association.

> Public health has its historical roots in the long recognized necessity of invoking governmental authority to protect the community against the spread of communicable disease. From these limited beginnings, the increasing interdependence of individuals living in a highly industrialized and urbanized society has brought major advances in both areas of governmental responsibility for individual well-being . . . Public health activities have increasingly entered

the area of services directly concerned with the personal health of individuals. With advances in medical science, the arbitrary line between prevention and treatment has narrowed and the distinction between community and individual health has become less sharply defined.[16]

The distinction between public health and preventive medicine is relevant to this conflict between public and private medicine. In general, public health refers to the organized efforts of society to control and prevent diseases that threaten the community as a whole. Preventive medicine differs from public health in its concern with the control and prevention of diseases that threaten the individual. While this distinction could be maintained to some degree in the era of communicable disease, it appears to make little sense in regard to the chronic, degenerative diseases. Increasingly coming into use is the term "medical care" as a more general term which, while traditionally referring to the care of individual patients, is coming more and more to stand for the overall organization of all medical services in the community.[17]

This controversy over medical care is presently centered around the issues of the economic costs and the adequacy and quality of such medical care. Various surveys of health needs and resources have revealed the unequal distribution of medical care among the different economic levels of our society. To help meet the need for medical care on the part of lower-income families in the face of rising medical costs, various health insurance plans have come into existence. The administration of these plans, the quality of care provided, and their effect upon other aspects of medical care such as hospital costs create some of the toughest problems in public health today. It seems inevitable that some form of tax-supported medical insurance plan will be established in the near future, but, as of the moment, this area provides one of the most heated controversies in public health.

These problems of delineation of responsibility and service areas are not mere academic disputations. They lie behind many of the current problems of providing adequate medical care and preventive services to all people; they lie at the heart of many of the current controversies and antagonisms among the different professionals in the field of medicine and public health; they present almost unsurmountable problems to collaboration in research, teaching, and service. To the sociologist with a concern for organizational structure and definitions of role and status, they offer many challenging areas for research. To the sociologist who wishes to make a career in the health field, they create many obstacles and frustrations.

Changing Needs in Public Health

The medical care system in the United States today is in a state of ferment. There can be little doubt that the entire field of public health will undergo many drastic changes in the next decade or two. This upheaval is the result of numerous economic, political, social, and medical forces. It reflects social changes in the composition of the population and the way people live. It represents a reaction of the public against the spiraling cost of medical care and a greater willingness to see the government play a more active role in the payment for medical services. It is the result of a changing disease picture and of rapid advances in medical knowledge. In general, so many social and medical changes have taken place in the past decade that it is little wonder that public health is experiencing a "cultural lag."

We conclude this chapter with a brief summary of some of the major trends in the field of health and medical care that have particular sociological relevance. The developments in the following listing are not mutually exclusive, since, for the most part, they are reflections of the same underlying social and medical forces. These developments may be classified into five main categories representing the different areas of major change in the public health picture today. Each has significant meaning for the future relationship of the behavioral sciences to problems of health and medical care.

A. Changes in the Nature of Disease

1. As the acute communicable diseases have been brought under control, there has been a corresponding increase in importance of the chronic degenerative diseases. Social factors are much more important for these latter diseases in etiology, treatment, and prevention. Specific infectious *agents* are being replaced by social and

psychological *processes* as "causes" of disease, while changes in one's way of life have become a crucial factor in the treatment of these chronic illnesses.

2. The age patterns of disease are changing with a shift in the vulnerable age groups from the young to the old. Older children and adolescents have given way to the middle-aged and the elderly, while concern with the intra-uterine child and the neonate is increasing.

3. The duration of illness is changing from the sudden and spectacular to the long-drawn-out and routine. The chronic diseases develop over many symptomless years and require long periods of continued care. Early detection and rehabilitation are becoming the symbols of modern public health.

B. *Changes in Social and Environmental Conditions*

1. Technological changes have produced new public health problems, such as air pollution, radiation, and food additives. The peaceful use of nuclear energy poses a real public health hazard. The automobile becomes an ever-increasing agent of death and disability.

2. The stress of modern living and the breakdown of social supports such as the family have increased the importance of mental illness as a public health problem. Alcoholism and narcotics addiction are also reflections of this trend.

3. The increased numbers of elderly people have created new public health demands for long-term care and special facilities. Home care and nursing homes are becoming increasingly important.

C. *Changes in Medical Care Practices and Organization*

1. The greater complexity of medical practice and the rapidity of new medical discoveries have increased the number of specialists, with a corresponding decrease in general practitioners. This has, in turn, created problems in the integration of medical services and in the continuity of care. Group practice or team medicine is offered as one possible answer to this problem.

2. The high cost of medical care has led to a rapid expansion of health insurance and increased pressure for some form of government-sponsored insurance plan.

3. There is a trend away from the hospital as the "workshop" of the physician to a more integrated position in community health as a whole. In the face of a shortage of hospital beds, many individuals are alarmed at the use of hospitals for custodial rather than medi-

cal care. There is a growing movement toward nursing homes and home care programs for such custodial care.

4. Medical welfare services are moving away from the "free public clinics" and are becoming an integral part of the organized governmental services provided to the indigent under public assistance funds. There is a great deal of current controversy about the quality of such medical care and the need for a more comprehensive approach to the problem.

5. Shortages in medical and nursing personnel have created serious problems of providing adequate care and have encouraged the development of quasi-medical personnel such as nurses' aides and dental assistants.

6. Medical education has become more costly and more complex. Medical schools are not turning out enough physicians to maintain the physician-population ratio and there is increasing demand for government support. The teaching of comprehensive medicine is being developed as an antidote to overspecialization. Courses in the behavioral sciences are gradually being introduced.

D. *Changes in Public Health Practice*

1. The prevention of illness is becoming more a matter of changing the habits and customs of individuals than controlling environmental conditions or immunizing populations. New methods of health education are needed to produce such changes in the behavior of individuals and customary practices of groups. Cultural differences among subgroups of the population require special attention.

2. The emphasis of public health upon legislation is giving way to a greater reliance upon voluntary participation. Many of the current sanitary measures have a stronger relationship to esthetics than to disease, and compliance has become a matter of public education and taste.

3. The initial emphasis of public health was upon establishing and providing services; today, with many such services in operation, the problem is becoming one of greater utilization. The public must now be motivated to make use of these services. Instead of waiting, these services must now develop techniques of "reaching out" to the public.

E. *Changes in Public Opinion and Behavior*

1. Health and happiness are being demanded by the public as a basic right rather than a privilege. People no longer expect and accept illness and early death as "natural." Medical care has

become a necessity of life and an essential part of any welfare program.
2. The public is taking a more active part in the determination of public health policy. The support of public opinion is becoming necessary both from the point of view of budgetary allocations to health departments and community support of voluntary health programs.
3. The public is showing a greater interest in medical matters, as evidenced by an increase in the number of health articles in lay publications and the growth of voluntary health agencies. The merchandising of drugs has become "big business," creating many problems of communication both for the public and for the medical profession.

These trends constitute a real challenge to traditional forms of public health activity. In addition to developing new programs to meet current health threats as they arise, local health departments are becoming increasingly involved in such administrative problems as the coordination of health services in a community and the provision of medical care to special subgroups of the population—the very young, the very old, the retarded, and the handicapped. In a rapidly changing society, it is not extraordinary that health and medical care should also be undergoing extensive modification. If these changes seem to be lagging somewhat, one must keep in mind the highly organized nature of medical services in the United States and the natural resistance of vested interests. It must also be remembered that the focus of our attention is upon social forces and these tend to become exaggerated through microscopic examination. Certainly, there is much in the everyday practice of the public health worker and physician that remains untouched, except in a theoretical sense, by the trends listed above. All is not problematical and there is a great deal to be accomplished by the traditional patterns of public health practice.

It should be apparent to the sociologist, from the list of developments in health and medical care presented above, that here, indeed, is an area of great relevance to the field of sociology. The remainder of this report will be devoted to indicating where and how the sociologist might bring his talents to bear upon these important social conditions and problems which also constitute medical and public health problems.

NOTES TO CHAPTER III

1. For a good introduction to the field of public health, the reader is referred to Hanlon, John J., *Principles of Public Health Administration*, 3d ed., C. V. Mosby Co., St. Louis, 1960. This volume contains two chapters dealing specifically with the behavioral sciences and social pathology.
2. Roney, James G., Jr., "Social Sciences in the Teaching of Public Health," *Journal of Health and Human Behavior*, vol. 1, Fall, 1960, p. 48.
3. Hanlon, John J., *op. cit.*, p. 140.
4. For a detailed description of the history of public health, the reader is referred to George A. Rosen's *A History of Public Health*, MD Publications, Inc., New York, 1958; F. H. Top's *The History of American Epidemiology*, C. V. Mosby Co., St. Louis, 1952; and John J. Hanlon's *Principles of Public Health Administration*, *op. cit.*, chaps. 1 and 2.
5. *Final Report of the Study Group on the Mission and Organization of the Public Health Service*. U.S. Dept. of Health, Education, and Welfare, Public Health Service, Washington, 1960.
6. California (Berkeley and Los Angeles), Columbia, Harvard, Johns Hopkins, Michigan, Minnesota, North Carolina, Pittsburgh, Puerto Rico, Tulane, and Yale.
7. The organization of mental health services is quite different from that of public health. Sometimes these programs are found within a public health department, and sometimes there is an entirely separate department of mental health. This report will be limited to public health services in general.
8. Greve, Clifford H., and Josephine R. Campbell, *Organization and Staffing for Local Health Services*. Rev. ed. U.S. Public Health Service, Publication No. 682, Government Printing Office, Washington, 1961, p. 1.
9. This guide is currently undergoing extensive revision. The APHA Committee on Public Health Administration is preparing three documents dealing with the evaluation of community health services: "Guide for a Study of Community Health Services," "Administration of Community Health Services," and "Indices of Community Health Services." The volume, *Administration of Community Health Services*, presents a comprehensive summary of current public health activities. (International City Managers' Association, Chicago, 1961.)
10. "The State Health Department-Services and Responsibilities: An Official Statement of the American Public Health Association," *American Journal of Public Health*, vol. 44, February, 1954, pp. 235–252.
11. Mountin, Joseph W., and Evelyn Flook, *Guide to Health Organization in the United States*. U.S. Public Health Service, Publication No. 196, Government Printing Office, Washington, 1953.
12. Hanlon, John J., *op. cit.*, p. 661.
13. Gunn, Selskar M., and Phillip S. Platt, *Voluntary Health Agencies:* An Interpretive Study. The Ronald Press Co., New York, 1945.
14. From a talk before the Eastern States Health Conference, April 27, 1961, New York City, on "Voluntary Action in the British Health Services."
15. Hamlin, Robert H., *Voluntary Health and Welfare Agencies in the United States*. The Schoolmasters' Press, New York, 1961, p. 3.
16. Editorial, "Tax-Supported Medical Care of the Needy," *American Journal of Public Health*, vol. 42, October, 1952, pp. 1314–1315.
17. For a comprehensive treatment of the organization and financing of medical care in the United States, the reader is referred to Somers, Herman M., and Anne R. Somers, *Doctors, Patients, and Health Insurance*, The Brookings Institution, Washington, 1961.

IV

SOCIOLOGY AND BASIC HEALTH PROCESSES

WE MAY DISTINGUISH four fundamental propositions affecting the relationship of sociology to public health:

1. Social factors are basic determinants in the distribution of many diseases. Disease is a phenomenon that varies geographically. Underlying these differential rates of occurrence are social and cultural conditions that strongly influence the disease environment of the individual—his exposure and his susceptibility.

2. Social factors play an important role in the etiology of many diseases. Such factors may act directly as causal agents in the occurrence of the disease or indirectly as contributing factors that increase or decrease the probability of disease.

3. Social factors define which health conditions shall be considered public health problems and the activities that may be carried out to meet these problems. The recognition of a disease as a threat to society, the allocation of responsibility, and the development of acceptable means for meeting this threat are functions of social control.

4. Social factors determine the response of society and the individual to many health problems. The meaning of illness, its perception and definition, and behavioral responses to illness are basic factors influencing the reactions of the public to public health programs.

These four generalizations, and the many corollaries that stem from them, constitute areas for basic social research in the field of health. The first proposition is firmly established in the traditional fields of medical ecology and demography. The second is rapidly achieving an accepted position with the increasing importance of the social epidemiology of the chronic diseases. The third is not as yet fully recognized as a fundamental challenge to the success of public health programs, except perhaps in underdeveloped areas where attempts at the rapid introduction of new approaches to health problems have forced a recognition of cultural factors in the acceptance and rejection of such public health activities. The fourth is growing in importance with the increased need for public cooperation in health programs and with the recognition of health behavior as social behavior. The remainder of this chapter will discuss these propositions in turn as they have given rise to four major areas of current social and public health research.

Ecology and Demography

Gregg, in a historical analysis of the development of public health, calls the present "an era of ecology" in which medical attention is slowly but surely shifting from a preoccupation with the disease entity to the study of the whole individual in his natural habitat.[1] The reason for this shift may be comprehended in part from the recognition that of the 19 leading causes of death today, only two represent conditions that can be controlled effectively by existing health measures.[2] The traditional approach to disease through isolation and control of the disease-causing agent must be supplemented by a greater understanding of man in relation to his total environment, social as well as physical.

According to the ecological approach, disease represents a maladjustment of the human organism to his environment. The disease process is initiated by a disturbance of the balance between man and nature. When this balance rests upon social forces in the environment, as it does for many of the chronic diseases and behavioral disorders, then *how* man lives becomes as important as *where* he lives in determining his state of health. The ecology of health, then, from a sociological point of view, becomes the study of the relationship between variations in man's social environment and his state of health.

The separation of man from his environment and, in turn, the social from the physical environment is, to a large extent, a matter of arbitrary distinction. Man is an inherent part of his own environment; he both shapes and is shaped by it. There is very little of the physical environment that is not altered by social or man-made conditions. The importance of these socioenvironmental conditions for man's health can be seen in the higher rates of disease, higher infant mortality, and lower life expectancy to be found in urban slums.[3] Much more than inadequate housing or unsanitary conditions is involved. Social pathology and health pathology are but different facets of the same social disorganization characterizing urban society.

Ecological comparisons between different areas showing high and low rates of disease according to the social characteristics of these areas have been used to identify possible social factors in disease. Thus Faris and Dunham, in one of the earliest ecological comparisons involving social factors, ascertained that high rates of first hospital admissions for a number of psychoses were to be found in areas of the city characterized by low socioeconomic status and high residential mobility.[4] Similar ecological comparisons have been made between neonatal mortality and the racial, ethnic, and income composition of census areas[5] and, on an international scale, between cardiovascular disease and dietary habits.[6]

While these ecological comparisons can produce worthwhile hypotheses for further etiological research, by themselves they cannot be taken as proof of a causal relationship or even an association between the factors being studied. As Robinson[7] and Clausen and Kohn[8] have pointed out, variations in rates of occurrence between phenomena in different areas do not necessarily mean that these phenomena are related. It is possible to have high ecological associations with little or no individual correlation.

The analysis of *demographic* variations in disease focuses upon the relationship between membership in different social groups and the occurrence of disease. Traditionally, public health has been concerned with differences in disease rates according to sex, age, and race.[9] More recently, health status surveys have begun to collect data on such additional sociological groupings as social class, education, occupation, marital status, and religion.[10] There is every reason to expect the trend toward the collection of more sociologically meaningful data to continue as such factors as family composition and organizational memberships are also investigated.

For the most part, sociological interpretation of demographic data on health and illness has been largely limited. This is probably due to the primary emphasis of such studies upon the computation of standardized incidence and prevalence rates rather than the explanation of why differences occur. These data serve as the basis for drawing up morbidity and mortality tables, making actuarial predictions of life expectancy, describing demographic changes in the composition of the population, and identifying groups with high and low risk of disease. One has only to compare the early population health surveys with those being conducted today to recognize the tremendous increase in concern with sociological variables for their own sake. The recent series of major studies conducted by the Commission on Chronic Illness represents a benchmark in greater demographic sophistication. These studies investigated a host of social group memberships, as well as such problems as the public's needs and utilization of medical resources for treatment and rehabilitation.[11]

One of the demographic variables receiving the greatest attention and which has proved to be as essential to an understanding of health as to social process is socioeconomic status. It should come as no surprise to the sociologist that large differences in the incidence of disease are to be found among different socioeconomic groups. As one of the major indicators of where and how people live, socioeconomic status could be expected to influence the entire disease process from exposure to disease-causing agents to ability to resist. However, of unexpected significance, as we shall see later, was the effect of socioeconomic status on the individual's definition of illness, his decision to seek medical care, his acceptability for treatment, the treatment he does receive, and his subsequent adjustment or rehabilitation. Also, it may be productive to "look behind" the observed differences in the occurrence of disease according to sex, age, race, and religion for similar sociological interpretations and implications.

Just a brief word can be said about one of the major areas of mutual sociological and public health concern related to demography—that of population growth and change. There is an interest, first, in the *rate* of growth and attempts to change this rate; second, in the *changing* nature of the population as it relates to health problems; and, third, in how populations move—the effect of *migration* upon health.

Population control is a major health problem in many areas of the world. This problem was officially recognized as a public health problem by the American Public Health Association, which issued the following policy statement:

> In many areas of the world, substantial population increase means malnutrition and outright starvation. In other areas, it may mean increased stress in family life, reduction of educational opportunity and the retardation of the industrial development on which a nation's rising standard of living depends. No problem—whether it be housing, education, food supply, recreation, communication, medical care—can be effectively solved if tomorrow's population increases out of proportion to the resources available to meet those problems.[12]

The statement then proceeds to call for an expansion of scientific research on: (a) all aspects of human fertility, and (b) the interplay of biological, psychological, and socioeconomic factors influencing population change. Several important social research studies have been made in Puerto Rico and elsewhere concerning the public acceptance or rejection of population control measures.[13] For the most part, these studies have documented the ill-effects of overpopulation upon health, but have shown the great difficulty in instituting planned efforts to control population growth. An excellent adaptation of sociological principles to the problem of family planning is offered by Bogue, who is currently conducting a series of social experiments on promoting birth control methods in Chicago.[14]

One of the most dramatic population changes taking place today involves the relative increase in the number of old people. Hauser and Shanas point out that during the 100 years between 1850 and 1950 the number of older persons increased eighteen-fold,[15] while the total population increased sixfold and the number of younger persons only fourfold. This increase has important social implications for public health. Disease patterns and the nature and extent of health problems are different for older people. Medical facilities and services, therefore, require adjustment to meet new demands. For example, the major emphasis of public health programs for the aged will have to shift from prevention to long-term treatment and rehabilitation.

Several sociological studies have concentrated upon the health needs of the aged as these relate to other social and psychological needs. A comprehensive survey by Kutner and associates has examined the role of old-age centers similar to well-baby centers under the auspices of health departments.[16] One of their main findings concerned the need to "reach out" to these old people instead of waiting for them to utilize health facilities. A study by Streib and his associates has concentrated upon the effect of occupational retirement in old age upon morbidity and mortality.[17] A nationwide study of the health needs of the older people has shown the intimate relationship between the social adjustment of the aged and their health.[18] The recent White House Conference on the Problems of the Aged brought together social scientists and medical and public health researchers in an attempt to study the problem of aging and to plan future research. Since health problems are an inherent aspect of old age, it is not surprising to find social gerontologists devoting a great deal of attention to the health of the aged.

One final aspect of the "geography of disease" deserving mention because of the closely overlapping interests of sociology and public health is migration. The movement of individuals from one area to another has important consequences for their social adjustment and health. This migration may involve internal shifts from rural to urban areas or external immigration from one country to another. Such movements may produce important changes not only in the individual's physical environment but also in his social and cultural milieux, and have been the subject of intensive investigation by sociologists and health researchers.

Studies in this area are too numerous to cite. Most of these studies have been descriptive in nature and have limited themselves to comparing the health status of migrants with nonmigrants, usually to the detriment of the migrant. The possibilities for a more theoretical approach are indicated by the following proposition underlying a current study of migration from a rural to an urban industrial area.

The process of socio-cultural change as manifested in migration from a rural to an urban industrial setting raises the probability of incongruity between the culture of the migrant and the social situation in which he lives. Such incongruities place excessive adjustive burdens on the social groups in which the migrant interacts and on the personality systems of individual migrants. Insofar as these stresses are not absorbed by small group systems and/or the personality system, recent migrants to the industrial city are likely to manifest increased rates of psychological, somatic, and social ill health.[19]

The emphasis of this analysis upon social process illustrates one of the main criticisms of much of the current research on ecology and demography—their lack of concern with theoretical formulations to explain the observed differences among geographical areas and social groups. To some extent, as we shall see next, this has been attempted in the field of social epidemiology.

Social Etiology of Disease

The search for the causes of disease is of primary importance to basic medical research. In the field of public health, one of the principal methods for investigating the causes of disease is epidemiology. In its broadest sense, epidemiology is human medical ecology. Disease is studied in terms of the mutual interaction and balance between the human individual as *host* to the disease, the infectious *agent* as the carrier of the disease, and the *environment* as the surrounding medium which affects both the resistance of the host and the virulence of the agent, and the contact between the two. Epidemiology is concerned with the study of variations in the occurrence of disease among different subgroups of the population—the discovery and description of these differences (descriptive epidemiology) and the analysis of the reasons for the differences (explanatory epidemiology). The basic method of epidemiology is the population survey.

From this brief description of epidemiology, it should be apparent to any social researcher that there is a strong kinship between the epidemiological survey and the social survey. When the objective of the research is to study the role of social factors in the etiology of disease, the two merge into what is known as social epidemiology. It is in this joining of social science focused on the definition and measurement of the independent variable—the social etiological factor—and medical science concerned with the identification and diagnosis of the disease state that perhaps the most fundamental wedding of sociology and public health can take place. With the steadily increasing importance of the chronic diseases and the behavioral disorders, the future of etiological medical research is inextricably bound up with the study of social factors. It is little wonder that this area of collaboration between the sociologist and the epidemiologist has been, and promises to continue to be, the most productive of significant research.

Social epidemiological surveys linking social factors with the occurrence of disease have been conducted for almost all the major chronic and behavioral disorders. It is understandable that the most extensive of these has been concerned with mental disease. Srole and his associates state as their most fundamental postulate: "Socio-cultural conditions, in both their normative and deviant forms, operating in intrafamily and extrafamily settings during childhood and adulthood have measurable consequences reflected in the mental health differences to be observed within a population."[20] Leighton and his associates are centering their attention on the role of social stress and social disorganization in mental health.[21] Hollingshead and Redlich have offered a detailed study of the relationship of social class to mental illness.[22] In other areas, large-scale social epidemiological studies have investigated the relationship of social factors to heart disease,[23] cancer,[24] and arthritis.[25] Many of these surveys would rank among the best of the social surveys, both methodologically and conceptually.

Fundamental to all of these surveys is the proposition that social factors play a significant role in the etiology of disease. While they vary greatly in the sophistication of their theoretical framework, in general, each views social factors within an open-system, rational model of multiple causality. According to this model, social factors are analyzed as only one part of a complex causal nexus in which no single factor is a necessary and sufficient explanation of the occurrence of the disease. The acceptance of an open-system, naturalistic, multi-causal model of illness and health as opposed to the closed-system, mechanistic, single-cause model of traditional medical and public health research is of basic importance to social epidemiological research. Dating from the discovery of bacteria, the closed-system model viewed each disease in terms of a single, specific cause which, ideally, would always produce the disease when present. Similarly, whenever any disease occurred, ideally, we would find a specific cause. In addition, a factor could be accepted as a cause only if it were directly related to the system primarily responsible for the disease symptoms.

Today we qualify causal factors with such adjectives as predisposing, contributory, and precipitating, and view the disease process as involving a multicausal network. Even within this network, furthermore, the reactions of any specific stimulus will depend upon other circumstances also being present. This reaction, in addition, may have as its antecedent a host of other stimuli or causes. The presence or absence of any of the circumstances under which the stimuli act become an essential part of the causal picture. Thus, we deal with the contribution of any single factor to the probability of disease rather than certainty. As Cornfield has pointed out,

> . . . the long and complicated chain between exposure to an agent and the subsequent development of the disease compels the consideration of probabilities and not certainties. The appropriate question to ask about agents in such situations is whether they alter the probability of an event's occurrence, and not whether they do or do not cause it.[26]

Social variables play their major role as such predisposing, contributing, and precipitating "causal" factors, and it is the determination of this role *in conjunction with the biological and physical* that constitutes the search for social factors as "causes" of disease. And, in a similar fashion, this open-system model is of basic importance to modern preventive public health. No longer can the public health worker seek, identify, and either destroy the agent or immunize the host in a simple, straightforward attack upon the single cause of a disease. Now, out of the myriad of complex, interrelated factors associated with a disease condition, he must locate those contributing factors that are, in the first place, capable of being manipulated and, in the second place, do not produce negative side-effects as the causal chain shifts to establish a new equilibrium when one of its components is disturbed. Furthermore, preventive action against any single contributing factor is likely to have only a small effect upon the total picture and results will tend to appear discouraging. Even when a number of factors can be controlled simultaneously, the public health worker probably must content himself with a proportionate reduction rather than the total elimination of a disease.

Thus whether one is willing to accept the proposition that social factors can cause disease, or that, in turn, disease can be controlled through the manipulation of social factors, depends largely upon one's concept of the etiology of disease. Most current formulations concerning the process through which social factors become related to disease hypothesize the social factors as affecting the disease state only indirectly either through stress situations that produce emotional reactions accompanied by physiological disturbances, or through environmental changes that increase the exposure and vulnerability of the individual or the progress of the disease process, or through changes in the individual himself that make him more susceptible to the disease. King gives an excellent summary of various theories that elucidate this process relating social factors to disease.[27]

In general, most current social epidemiological studies are deficient in the conceptualization of their social variables and in the development of a theory as to how and why the social factors become engaged in the disease process. Many public health epidemiologists are content to limit their research to the simple discovery of significant differences in the occurrence of disease among different social groups. However, as in the case of the social survey, these observed differences must be taken as only the jumping-off place in a search for underlying factors that will help to explain why the differences occur. The latent meaning of the statistical categories as indicative of meaningful social groups within the community, and as representative of different group organizations, values, and ways of living must be explored. Sex, age, occupation, marital status, and economic class differences in health status take on added meaning in terms of differing sex and age roles and statuses, exposure to occupational stress, family relationships, social class mobility, and so forth. Just as the social researcher takes these group differences as only indirect measures of social behavior, so must the public health researcher translate these static group differences into a dynamic analysis of the process whereby group memberships can affect the causes and consequences of disease.

In one of the most comprehensive attempts to integrate social factors into the disease sequence, Caudill postulates an interdependence between the social and the biological so that a strain on one involves an adaptation of the other.[28] The future need insofar as mental illness is concerned is described by Clausen as involving the development of social and psychological theory that deals with the relationship of the individual to society and the way in which a disruption of this relationship may result in physical or mental illness.[29]

In our opinion, the future development of public health programs to cope with the increasingly serious spread of the chronic diseases and behavioral disorders will be greatly aided by an extensive exchange of concepts, theories, and methods between sociology and epidemiology. Epidemiology is the basic tool of public health research but it currently lacks a theoretical framework for deriving hypotheses and for interpreting research findings involving social factors. Epidemiology may well have to borrow, adopt, and then modify large segments of sociological theory concerning individual and group behavior.

Furthermore, epidemiology may be able to profit from the research experience sociology has had with laboratory experiments involving social groups and with controlled experiments in natural settings. It may not be too far fetched to imagine that the most prevalent public health problems in the future will require research that involves the manipulation of a large number of socio-environmental factors for very large samples. These problems will require a broad focus upon all factors affecting the human organism, biological and social. In one sense, the chronic diseases and behavioral disorders are progressive and cumulative in etiology, and everything that impinges upon the individual may affect the probability of his developing any of these diseases.

In summary, we might say that there is such a close relationship between social epidemiology and sociology that it might almost be valid to characterize it as "public health sociology."

The Determination and Control of Health Problems

Numerous anthropological studies bear witness to the fact that what is regarded as a serious health problem in one society may be considered "normal" in another. The acceptability of health innovations in underdeveloped areas has been found to depend a great deal upon the culture's recognition of the innovation as being a "practical" way of meeting a felt health need. Thus, for example, in Peru, the use of hot water among Indians was appropriate only in households where someone was sick; in Puerto Rico, attempts to introduce contraceptive measures for birth control conflicted with the society's definition of male virility and authority over women; in India, caste obligations that bound the villager to the faith healer interfered with efforts to introduce medical professionals. Numerous such examples are given by Polgar in his extensive review of the literature.[30]

As Parsons has indicated, medicine constitutes an important subsystem in American society. This system of health care reflects the basic value orientation and social organization of the larger society.[31] Sigerist has pointed out that the place of medicine in a society is determined by the current social and economic structure, the valuation that society places on health and disease, the tasks assigned to its physicians, and the technology of medicine available to doctors at the time.[32] Modern culture places great emphasis upon scientific medicine as opposed to folk or primitive medicine. Sociocultural forces play a large part in determining the meaning of illness—when a person can legitimately claim to be ill; the functions of illness—the changes in his behavior that are acceptable as a result of the illness; and the ways of counteracting illness—the preventive and therapeutic measures that may be used to fight illness.

The need for public health workers to take these sociocultural factors into account in planning and developing health services has been illustrated by a series of case studies edited by Paul.[33] The way culture can affect the acceptability of health services is illustrated by Paul in discussing the role of beliefs and customs for sanitation programs.

> In parts of Latin America, maternity patients of moderate means expect a private hospital room with an adjoining alcove to accommodate a servant or kinswoman who comes along to attend the patient around the clock. In parts of rural India, the hospital should be built with a series of separate cooking stalls where the patient's family can prepare the meals, in view of cultural prohibitions against the handling of food by members of other castes. And, of course, the effect of cultural differences looms even larger where sanitation has to be built directly into the habit systems of people, rather than into structures and plants that serve the people.[34]

Wellin has stated that the implication of culture for health activities involves two fundamental questions: How does the community perceive and respond to the health program? How do health workers perceive and respond to the community and its culture?[35] In an excellent review of the social factors affecting public health activities, Foster discusses various cultural barriers to new public health programs that stem from a society's value system regarding health, such as (1) suspicion of new things; (2) fatalism; (3) conflict with religious values; and (4) dysfunctional social structure.[36]

That the goals and means of public health represent, to a large extent, the dominant aims and values of a society has been pointed out by a number of medical historians. As Hanlon and his associates describe the development of a philosophy of public health, each period of history may be seen to have had its own ideal of what constituted public health. The goals of public health are found to represent the prevailing religious, economic, and social values of any particular period. Thus the recognition and acceptance of mental health as a public health problem could not take place so long as the concept of health was limited by the theological concept of sin.[37]

An excellent current illustration of a conflict in values concerning a public health problem is afforded by the controversy over the best approach to the control of traffic accidents, one of the major causes of death and disability today. Involved are conflicting values of public safety versus personal convenience; of streamlined, speedy vehicles versus slower vehicles with protective devices; of the rights of pedestrians versus those of the drivers. The importance of social values in determining public action in this area was highlighted at a recent conference on passenger car design and highway safety.[38]

This discussion of public health activities in terms of social values highlights the fact that, in large measure, public health problems are social problems. The social forces that determine whether a health condition will be viewed as a public health problem are similar to those that define a social problem in general. To some extent, it is not incorrect to attribute much of the origin of the modern public health movement to early attempts of social reformers to meet the social problems created by the industrial revolution and the rise of the urban slum. As Dubos states, "Out of the reform efforts of the nineteenth century, there emerged our modern concepts of sanitation and public health."[39]

From this viewpoint, the sociological formulations concerning the nature of social problems are directly applicable to an understanding of public health problems. For example, according to the formulation developed by Merton and Nisbet, we may view many public health problems as "the unwilled, largely indirect, and often unanticipated consequences of institutionalized patterns of social behavior." Certainly this is true of many of the communicable and chronic diseases arising from urbanization and the stresses of modern living. Of particular interest to us in the present context of defining public health activities is Merton's and Nisbet's analysis of the way in which conflicts in values hamper public policies designed to solve social problems.[40]

Thus many current controversies in public health concerning such issues as fluoridation, radiation, air pollution, accident prevention, use of insecticides, alcoholism, and narcotics addiction are bound to be fought in the arena of public opinion and conflicting special interests. The role of special interest groups in defining public health problems is vividly characterized in the following statement concerning dietary problems in the control of heart disease: "Having only recently emerged scarred and nonvictorious from the battlefield of cigarette smoking versus cancer of the lung, I can testify that the dairy and beef trusts, as well as the hamburger and custard stands, will not willingly give up their vested and powerful interests."[41] Whether or not an undesirable social condition will be perceived as a public health problem, to a large extent, will depend upon the public image of that problem and its willingness to relegate responsibility to public health authority. Thus, at the moment, narcotics addiction is primarily regarded as a legal problem and only recently have public health and medical professionals challenged this definition.

It has been maintained that the public gets the kind of health programs it demands or deserves. We see this in the continued operation of public health programs that no longer represent the best professional judgment, as in the case of public anxiety supporting the overinstitutionalization of the mentally ill or the public's support of an outmoded restaurant inspection system, and in the inability of public health departments to initiate new programs such as fluoridation or accident prevention.

The relationship of health problems to social problems can be dealt with only briefly here. Many public health problems are social problems and vice versa. Alcoholism, venereal disease, mental illness, narcotics addiction are common ground for public health workers and sociologists alike. Both their manifestations and consequences are rooted in social processes, and the values attached to them by society define these "social diseases" as social problems. Part of the difficulty public health meets in trying to deal with these problems is the public's reluctance to view them as medical problems. The social stigma attached to these diseases creates serious problems of case-finding and prevention. Conversely, the reluctance of the public health field to view these health problems as social problems has often resulted in the failure of public health programs aimed at their control.

In turn, such social problems as juvenile delinquency, divorce, housing, and such major social developments as urbanization, population growth, increased numbers of old people are important factors in many current public health problems. These common problems constitute a natural arena for combined public health and sociological research. Changes in the demographic composition of our population, in the growth of cities and suburbs, in the solidarity of the family, in the values and morals of young people, all give rise to significant public health problems that can best be dealt with through an attack on their social origins.

The relationship between social problems and health problems may be viewed as a reversible one. On the one hand, social problems may lead to health problems as in the case of slum housing leading to disease, while, on the other hand, health problems may create social problems as in the case of the venereal diseases When we further introduce the concept of social values affecting the legitimacy of the social or medical problem as "acceptable and appropriate" for corrective action, we find that we may hypothesize four types of social and health problems as illustrated in the following chart:

	Social Acceptability	
	Acceptable	Not Acceptable
Social Problem→Health Problem	A	B
Health Problem→Social Problem	C	D

Type A would represent those social problems that create health conditions, both of which are acceptable to society. An example would be mental illness that resulted from some such acceptable social process as overwork, or a personal or family calamity. Type B would reflect the same process but in an area of social disapproval, such as juvenile delinquency leading to an increase in venereal disease. An example of Type C, a health problem that results in a social problem, both acceptable, would be some crippling injury sustained as the result of an accident that leads to unemployment, while Type D, both unacceptable, would be represented by alcoholism leading to divorce or crime.

Wolff has used the term "social pathology" to describe this relation between disease and social conditions,[42] a term adopted by Hanlon to signify "a state of community imbalance evidenced by significant prevalence of disease and its related social disorders."[43] The so-called "social diseases" are prime examples of social pathology. From a sociological point of view, we may view these social diseases as socially disapproved health conditions that are usually brought about by the individual's own deviant behavior. Rather than the sick individual being the unfortunate victim of some chance infection, he is thought to have brought about his own ill health; thereafter to be condemned and perhaps punished rather than pitied and cared for.

Merton's analysis of the social and cultural factors in deviant behavior is particularly appropriate to the study of these social diseases. It becomes extremely important to "discover how some social structures exert a definite pressure upon certain persons in the society to engage in nonconforming rather than conforming conduct."[44] This approach to public health problems in terms of deviant behavior has been found to be particularly appropriate to the study of disorders such as alcoholism and narcotics addiction.[45] Clausen views the use of narcotics as only one possible manifestation of social disorganization and emphasizes the need to approach drug addiction as part of a whole series of social-health problems.[46] Alcoholism and narcotics addiction are also good examples of health conditions in which the demand for public health action stems not from the medical condition itself but rather from the antisocial behavior of its victims.

Finally, we would like to mention briefly the social effects of disease as an area where sociology has a natural contribution to make to public health. Diseases not only have social causes; they have social consequences as well. These effects may be felt by the society as a whole, as in the case of a widespread epidemic; by the group, such as the family of a chronic invalid; or by the sick individual himself. History is full of examples of the profound effects that epidemics have had upon whole societies. Changes in the birth and death rates have widespread implications for the kinds of social, economic, and political problems a nation will have to face. Foote and Cottrell[47] have indicated some of the ways in which health constitutes an important component of interpersonal competence.

Public health action itself may have many direct and indirect social effects. Indeed, one might say that the purpose of public health is to change the society within which it operates. Successful public health programs in population control, for example, will have profound social consequences comparable to those of other successful public health programs, such as those resulting in malaria control and immunization against the communicable diseases of childhood, which have changed the face of the society in which we live today. The decrease in infant death rates and an increase in longevity produce increased need for schools for the young and housing for the aged.

While the study of the social consequences of disease would appear to be an excellent area for sociological research, relatively little work has been done that views illness as the independent variable and its effects as the dependent variable. When one considers the pervasive nature of illness, and its importance in the life of the individual, the study of the impact of illness should provide a challenging area for the testing of sociological hypotheses concerning human behavior in crisis situations.

Social Responses to Health Problems

How an individual reacts to the threat of personal illness and how a community responds to a public health problem are basic questions in medical sociology. In this final section, we will examine some of the more fundamental theoretical issues involved in understanding social behavior in relation to health problems, reserving a discussion of the application of these general principles to specific public health programs for the next chapter.

Illness is a social phenomenon. It occurs in all societies and is defined and fought in terms of the particular cultural forces prevalent in a society. As many ethnographic studies have shown, different societies have developed characteristic ways of dealing with illness. The values and customs of a community or a social group strongly influence their perception of the symptoms of disease, their interpretation of these symptoms, and their techniques for treatment. This has been found to be the case even within our own culture where several studies have shown that different social classes and different ethnic and religious groups respond differently to illness and to health programs. Members of the lower socioeconomic groups are less likely to utilize existing health facilities or to take part in preventive health programs. Hollingshead and Redlich found that diagnosis and treatment for mental illness was a function of class membership.[48] Deasy has demonstrated how variations in socioeconomic level affected the proportion of mothers who had their children immunized against poliomyelitis.[49] Koos provides ample evidence that social class membership affected the perception and interpretation of symptoms.[50] Thus, it would seem, while death may level all ranks and stations, illness serves only to exaggerate social class differences.

From a sociological point of view, there are extremely significant differentiations to be made between the concepts of disease, illness, and sickness. It is interesting to note the following definition of disease in a purely physiological textbook: "Health and disease are primarily sociological concepts; they generally mean that a man can or cannot carry on his normal occupation."[51] This accent on functioning is a valid one and is basic to the determination of illness. In the case of physiological functioning, we have developed more standardized measures of "health" than is true for mental or social functioning, although, as the World Health Organization points out, "Health then may be expressed as a degree of conformity to accepted standards of given criteria in terms of basic conditions of age, sex, community and region, within normal limits of variation."[52] Health is thus a relative concept and subject to social as well as medical interpretation.

The important point to be recognized here is that the way people define illness and the way they respond to it and to public health attempts at prevention, treatment, and rehabilitation will depend a great deal upon their social group memberships. Zborowski has even shown that cultural factors affect the perception of and response to pain.[53]

It might be productive to distinguish between *disease* as referring to the medical entity, defined in terms of biological or physiological functioning; *illness* as the social entity or status, defined in terms of social functioning; and *sickness* as the personal reactions of the individual, defined in terms of his own feeling state and the reactions of others toward his illness. Thus we commonly speak of the disease *process*, the *condition* of illness, and the sick *role*. Two persons with the same disease process can have different degrees of illness and different degrees and types of sickness; also, persons with the same disease process and the same condition of illness can have different degrees and types of sickness.

The significant research question for public health becomes when and how is the presence of a disease as diagnosed by the medical specialist defined as an illness by the group, and how do these processes relate to the patient's feelings toward the disease and the state of being sick. Certainly, the study of responses to public health programs must take into account these differences between professional, group, and individual perceptions of disease and illness.

A recent analysis by King has shown how these variations in the perception of illness on the part of patients can be traced to the influence of a wide range of factors upon the way people perceive objects and situations in general. These factors range from biochemical agents and constitutional factors through personality and character variables to social status, role, and cultural values and beliefs. King also points out that the health professionals' beliefs and perceptions about illness will exert an influence upon their own behavior in relation to the public and to other professionals.[54]

An area that has received a great deal of sociological attention is medical behavior as a social act. The definition and recognition of illness, the seeking of medical care, and the response to treatment are forms of social behavior. As such, there is a great deal that the sociologist can contribute to an understanding of how individuals and groups behave in the face of a health problem. This was clearly recognized by Parsons in his development of the concept of a "sick role" to characterize the behavior of the sick individual. The ill person is usually someone who is exempted from his normal social responsibilities; he is not held morally responsible for being ill but he is obligated to try to get well as quickly as possible. He must seek medical care as a "legitimatization" of his sick status, but the doctor-patient relationship contains many complications both for him and for the doctor. "The strains existing on *both* sides of a doctor-patient relationship are such that we must expect to find, not merely institutionalization of the roles, but special mechanisms of social control in operation."[55]

Other social scientists have challenged Parsons' concept of illness as a form of "deviant" behavior—for example, inability of the sick individual to meet his task and role demands—and have attempted to show the importance of the individual's social group membership upon his behavior in seeking and responding to medical care. The behavior of an ill person seeking medical care is described by Caudill as follows:

> In his own experience, an individual with a physical illness is likely to feel its effect in the psychological processes of his personality, and also to turn to his family for emotional and other support. If the family is nonexistent or disrupted, he may turn to other small groups such as his friends, or seek greater emotional support than is usually expected in his relations with his personal physician, pastor, or employer. It is at this point, and beyond, that the more overt cultural differences in values, patterns of help and support, and social organization will strongly influence his behavior. If his more immediate sources of help are not satisfactory, he may turn to organized community aid through clinics, social agencies, and so on.[56]

Freidson makes an interesting distinction between the "professional referral structure" and the "lay referral structure." The professional referral structure he defines as a network of hierarchical *medical* relationships; the lay referral structure he describes as follows:

> Indeed, the whole process of seeking help involves a network of potential consultants, from the intimate and informal confines of the nuclear family through successively more select, distant, and authoritative laymen, until the "professional" is reached. This network of consultants, which is part of the structure of the local lay community and which imposes form on the seeking of help, might be called the "lay referral structure." Taken together with the cultural understandings involved in the process, we may speak of it as the "lay referral system."[57]

The sociology of the sick individual is becoming an area of increasing interest among sociologists, and the knowledge gained from social research on the behavior of the ill should prove very valuable to public health, especially in relation to prevention of disease through early diagnosis, utilization of health services, and adjustment to and rehabilitation of chronic conditions. A current research project by the New York City Department of Health is attempting to study the different stages that characterize the pattern of behavior in regard to illness. This project hypothesizes five stages as follows:

1. The symptom experience stage: when the symptoms are (a) recognized, (b) interpreted as to their seriousness, possible cause, and

their import or meaning, (c) reacted to with varying degrees of concern.

2. The sick seeking status stage: when the potentially ill person begins to seek symptom alleviation, information and advice, and provisional validation from family, friends, or other nonprofessionals (the lay referral structure).

3. The medical contact stage: when one or more sources of medical care are contacted to ascertain a diagnosis and discover what courses of treatment will be recommended (the professional referral structure).

4. The dependent-patient role stage: when the individual has committed himself into the hands of a doctor, surrendered certain prerogatives and decisions, and accepted care.

5. The rehabilitation stage: when the individual returns to his normal role functioning.[58]

In an analysis of the relationship of sociocultural factors to responses to illness, Suchman has shown that membership in social groups that may be characterized as "cosmopolitan" is highly related to a "scientific" approach to health and medical care, while membership in "parochial" groups is more likely to lead to a "popular" or "folk" approach. The nature of this sociomedical health orientation is found to underly the individual's knowledge, attitudes, and behavior regarding illness and medical care. To the extent that the individual belongs to cosmopolitan social groups that share a scientific orientation to health and medical care, it is predicted, conflict with medical and public health professionals will be at a minimum.[59]

Other studies in this area are being conducted by Reader at Cornell in an attempt to determine the pattern of interpersonal expectations descriptive of the sick role in ambulatory patients with long-term illness, and by Barker at the University of Kansas in an attempt to study the psychological ecology of sickness. The latter project is investigating the social-psychological aspects of children's illness in a midwest town through a study of the incidence of illness and its consequences for the behavior of those closely involved; that is, the patient, his family, and the medical profession, with emphasis on the meaning of sickness as a physical and social fact to these classes of persons, and disparities in meaning that may impair the effectiveness of the medical services available.

The adjustment stage following illness has been the subject of several sociological studies, especially in relation to heart disease and mental health. Public health has yet to meet the problem of aftercare for mental patients discharged from hospitals and returning to the community. This transition is likely to be a crucial one, and is being studied by the Harvard University School of Public Health in an attempt to identify the significant variables in the post-hospital experience of mental patients, and to specify the relationship between these variables as they affect the rehabilitative process.

It is perhaps in this rapidly expanding area of rehabilitation that we find most current public health interest in the long-term effects of illness. As described by Rusk:

> We now talk about the third phase of medical care, the first being obviously prevention, the second, definitive medicine and surgery, and the third, that phase between the bed and the job—what you do after the fever is down and the stitches are out to allow the chronically ill or the physically disabled person to lead a self-supporting, self-respecting life with dignity.[60]

Public health agencies are beginning to play an increasingly greater role in the problem of rehabilitation for the chronically ill and the physically handicapped. It is well known that a physical disability may have tremendous effects upon the social and psychological outlook of the handicapped person. Richardson and his associates have done some interesting research on the self-image of the handicapped child. A Social Science Research Council bulletin, *Adjustment to Physical Handicap and Illness*, deals in great detail with the problem of adjustment and the effects of the handicap upon the individual.[61]

These studies of the behavior of individuals regarding illness are, of course, fundamental to the planning and operation of public health programs. As we shall see in the next chapter, the principles governing medical behavior are directly applicable to public participation in mass detection, immunization, treatment, and rehabilitation programs. Early detection of disease is particularly crucial for the chronic diseases and an increasing portion of public health work is devoted to mass screening programs. However, detection is only the first step and, to be effective, such programs must also induce individuals with positive findings to seek medical care. Here we run into a second crucial problem of public health work—the utilization of facilities. Finally, since many disabilities are not curable, it is necessary to provide for the adjustment or rehabilitation of the sick individual, and once again, an understanding of social behavior becomes essential. Thus we see that social responses to health problems affect all three stages of public health work—primary, secondary, and tertiary prevention.

NOTES TO CHAPTER IV

1. Gregg, Alan, "The Future Health Officer's Responsibility: Past, Present, and Future," *American Journal of Public Health*, vol. 46, 1956, pp. 1384–1389.
2. James, George, "Community Disease Detection Programs," *New York State Journal of Medicine*, vol. 61, August 15, 1961, p. 2757.
3. Anderson, Odin W., "Infant Mortality and Social and Cultural Factors" in Jaco, E. Gartly, editor, *Patients, Physicians and Illness*. The Free Press, Glencoe, Ill., 1958, pp. 10–23.
4. Faris, Robert E. L., and Warren H. Dunham, *Mental Disorders in Urban Areas*. University of Chicago Press, Chicago, 1939.
5. Willie, Charles, and William B. Rothney, "Racial, Ethnic and Income Factors in the Epidemiology of Neonatal Mortality," *American Sociological Review*, vol. 27, August, 1962, pp. 522–526.
6. Keys, Ancel, "The Diet and the Development of Coronary Heart Disease," *Journal of Chronic Diseases*, vol. 4, October, 1956, pp. 364–380.
7. Robinson, William D., "Ecological Correlations and the Behavior of Individuals," *American Sociological Review*, vol. 15, June, 1950, pp. 351–357.
8. Clausen, John A., and Melvin L. Kohn, "The Ecological Approach in Social Psychiatry," *American Journal of Sociology*, vol. 60, September, 1954, pp. 140–151.
9. United States National Office of Vital Statistics, *Health and Demography*. U.S. Public Health Service, Publication No. 502, Government Printing Office, Washington, October, 1956.
10. United States Public Health Service, *Origin and Program of the U.S. National Health Survey*. Publication No. 584-A1, Government Printing Office, Washington, May, 1958. The reports are divided into two series: A deals with methodological problems while B presents substantive findings.
11. See reports by Commission on Chronic Illness, *Chronic Illness in the United States*, Harvard University Press, Cambridge, 1955–1959, vols. 1–4.
12. *The New York Times*, November 19, 1959, p. 41.
13. Stycos, Mayone J., "Birth Control Clinics in Crowded Puerto Rico" in Paul, Benjamin D., editor, *Health, Culture, and Community*. Russell Sage Foundation, New York, 1955, pp. 189–210.
14. Bogue, Donald J., "Some Tentative Recommendations for a Sociologically Correct Family Planning Communication and Motivation Program in India." (To be published in a volume on world fertility by the Princeton University Press.)
15. Hauser, Philip M., and Ethel Shanas, "Trends in the Ageing Population" in Lansing, Albert I., editor, *Cowdry's Problems of Ageing*. Williams and Wilkins Co., Baltimore, 1952, pp. 966–968.

16. Kutner, Bernard, and associates, *Five Hundred Over Sixty*. Russell Sage Foundation, New York, 1956.
17. Streib, Gordon, Wayne Thompson, and Edward A. Suchman, "The Cornell Study of Occupational Retirement," *Journal of Social Issues*, vol. 14, no. 2, 1958, pp. 3–17. See entire issue.
18. Shanas, Ethel, "Some Findings from a National Study of the Health Needs of Older People," *Proceedings* of the Joint Council to Improve the Health Care of the Aged, Washington, D. C., June, 1959.
19. Cassel, John, Ralph Patrick, and David Jenkins, "Epidemiological Analysis of the Health Implications of Culture Change: A Conceptual Model," *Annals of the New York Academy of Sciences*, vol. 84, art. 17, December, 1960, p. 944.
20. Srole, Leo, and others, *Mental Health in the Metropolis*. McGraw-Hill Book Co., New York, 1962, p. 13.
21. Leighton, Alexander, *My Name Is Legion*. Basic Books, Inc., New York, 1959. See also *Interrelations Between the Social Environment and Psychiatric Disorders:* 1952 Annual Conference of the Milbank Memorial Fund, Milbank Memorial Fund, New York, 1953.
22. Hollingshead, August B., and Frederick C. Redlich, *Social Class and Mental Illness*. John Wiley and Sons, New York, 1958.
23. Dawber, Thomas R., and others, "Some Factors Associated with the Development of Coronary Artery Disease," *American Journal of Public Health*, vol. 49, October, 1959, pp. 1349–1356.
24. Wynder, E. L., and others, "A Study of Environmental Factors in Carcinoma of the Cervix," *American Journal of Obstetrics and Gynecology*, vol. 68, 1954, pp. 1016–1047.
25. Cobb, Sidney, and others, "An Estimate of the Prevalence of Rheumatoid Arthritis," *Journal of Chronic Diseases*, vol. 5, June, 1957, pp. 636–643.
26. Cornfield, Jerome, "Principles of Research," *American Journal of Mental Deficiency*, vol. 64, September, 1959, pp. 242–252.
27. King, Stanley H., "Social Psychological Factors in Illness" in Freeman, Howard, Sol Levine, and Leo G. Reeder, editors, *Handbook of Medical Sociology*. Prentice-Hall, Inc., Englewood Cliffs, N. J., 1963, pp. 99–121.
28. Caudill, William, *Effects of Social and Cultural Systems in Reactions to Stress*. Social Science Research Council, Pamphlet 14, New York, 1958. See also Simmons, Leo W., and Harold G. Wolff, *Social Science in Medicine*, Russell Sage Foundation, New York, 1954.
29. Clausen, John A., *Sociology and the Field of Mental Health*. Russell Sage Foundation, New York, 1956, p. 19. This review presents a good summary of research on the relationship between social stress and mental disorder.
30. Polgar, Steven, "Health and Human Behavior: Areas of Interest Common to the Social and Medical Sciences," *Current Anthropology*, vol. 3, April, 1962, pp. 159–205.
31. Parsons, Talcott, *The Social System*. The Free Press, Glencoe, Ill., 1951. See also Parsons' "Definitions of Health and Illness in the Light of American Values and Social Structure" in Jaco, E. Gartly, editor, *op. cit.*, pp. 165–187.
32. Sigerist, Henry E., "Place of Physician in Modern Society," *Proceedings of the American Philosophical Society*, vol. 90, 1946, pp. 275–279.
33. Paul, Benjamin D., editor, *Health, Culture, and Community:* Case Studies of Public Reaction to Health Programs. Russell Sage Foundation, New York, 1955.
34. Paul, Benjamin D., "The Role of Beliefs and Customs in Sanitation Programs," *American Journal of Public Health*, vol. 48, November, 1958, p. 1502.
35. Wellin, Edward, "Implications of Local Culture for Public Health," *Human Organization*, vol. 16, Winter, 1958, pp. 16–18.
36. Foster, George M., *Problems in Intercultural Health Programs*. Social Science Research Council, Pamphlet 12, New York, 1958.

37. Hanlon, John J., Fred B. Rogers, and George Rosen, "A Bookshelf on the History and Philosophy of Public Health," *American Journal of Public Health*, vol. 50, April, 1960, pp. 445–458. This bibliography provides a comprehensive list of readings on the historical development and current state of public health.
38. Monto, Alexander V., "Discussion" in *Passenger Car Design and Highway Safety*. Association for the Aid of Crippled Children and Consumer's Union of U.S., Inc., New York, 1962, p. 20.
39. Dubos, René J., "Beyond Traditional Medicine," *The Crisis in American Medicine*. A special supplement to *Harper's Magazine*, October, 1960, p. 168.
40. Merton, Robert K., and Robert A. Nisbet, editors, *Contemporary Social Problems*. Harcourt, Brace and World, Inc., New York, 1961.
41. Spain, David M., "Problems in the Study of Coronary Atherosclerosis in Population Groups," *Annals of the New York Academy of Sciences*, vol. 84, December 8, p. 831.
42. Wolff, George, "Social Pathology as a Medical Science," *American Journal of Public Health*, vol. 42, December, 1952, pp. 1576–1582.
43. Hanlon, John J., *Principles of Public Health Administration*. 3d ed. C. V. Mosby Co., St. Louis, 1960.
44. Merton, Robert K., *Social Theory and Social Structure*. Rev. ed. The Free Press, Glencoe, Ill., 1957, p. 132.
45. Suchman, Edward A., "The Addictive Disorders as Socio-Environmental Health Problems" in Freeman, Levine, and Reeder, editors, *op. cit.*, pp. 123–143.
46. Clausen, John A., "Drug Addiction" in Merton, Robert K., and Robert A. Nisbet, editors, *op. cit.*, pp. 194–195.
47. Foote, Nelson N., and Leonard S. Cottrell, Jr., *Identity and Interpersonal Competence*. University of Chicago Press, Chicago, 1955.
48. Hollingshead, August B., and Frederick C. Redlich, *op. cit.*
49. Deasy, Leila C., "Socioeconomic Status and the Poliomyelitis Vaccine Trial," *American Sociological Review*, vol. 21, April, 1956, p. 185.
50. Koos, Earl L., *The Health of Regionville*. Columbia University Press, New York, 1954.
51. Winton, F. R., and L. E. Bayliss, *Human Physiology*. 4th ed. Little, Brown, and Co., Boston, 1955, p. 1.
52. World Health Organization, *Measurements of Levels of Health*. Technical Report Series No. 137, Geneva, 1957, pp. 8–10.
53. Zborowski, Mark, "Cultural Components in Responses to Pain," *Journal of Social Issues*, vol. 8, 1952, pp. 16–30.
54. King, Stanley H., *Perceptions of Illness and Medical Practice*. Russell Sage Foundation, New York, 1962.
55. Parsons, Talcott, *The Social System*, p. 450. (See note 31.)
56. Caudill, William, *op. cit.*, p. 27.
57. Freidson, Eliot, "Client Control and Medical Practice," *American Journal of Sociology*, vol. 65, 1960, p. 377. For a good analysis of factors in patient's choice of medical service, see also Freidson's *Patients' Views of Medical Practice*, Russell Sage Foundation, New York, 1961.
58. Gilliam, Sylvia, "Role Dominance and Patterns of Medical Care." Paper read at the 1959 Annual Meeting of the American Sociological Association.
59. Suchman, Edward A., "Social Patterns in Health and Medical Care." Paper read at the 1963 Annual Meeting of the American Sociological Association.
60. Rusk, Howard, "America's Number One Medical Problem," *Proceedings* of the 42nd Annual Meeting of the Life Insurance Association of America, December 9, 1948, p. 58. A concise summary of the extent of the rehabilitation problem can be found in Rusk, H., and F. Taylor, "Physical Disability: A National Problem," *American Journal of Public Health*, vol. 38, October, 1948, pp. 1381–1386.
61. *Adjustment of Physical Handicap and Illness*. Social Science Research Council, Bulletin 55, rev. ed., New York, 1953.

V

SOCIOLOGY APPLIED TO PUBLIC HEALTH PRACTICE

THE DAILY ACTIVITIES of public health practitioners consist largely of the highly pragmatic operation of numerous public health programs. While the field of public health in its growth toward professional status has shown increasing interest in understanding the social processes discussed in the previous chapter, the primary concern of public health is still what it should be— the devising and carrying out of action programs to meet the health needs of the public. This field of public health practice is largely based upon practical personal experience and only recently have attempts been made to codify some of the more general principles of program operation into a branch of administrative science.

The conduct of public health programs requires to a large extent a combination of medical knowledge about the nature of disease, administrative knowledge concerning the organization, staffing, and operation of public health facilities, and social science knowledge dealing with community forces and individual behavior. The focus of this chapter will be upon the contribution that sociology has to make in supplying useful knowledge and techniques to the public health practitioner in his attempts to secure the support and cooperation of the public. The need to take social factors into account in the planning, development, and operation of public health programs is well recognized by the public health profession. As stated in an editorial in the *American Journal of Public Health:*

> Health workers agree generally that we are now in a period when the human factor must be taken into account if public health is to handle its problems successfully. Many of the areas of health with

which public health is today concerned involve individual voluntary action on the part of many people. There is also an increasing awareness that attitudes, beliefs, motives affect the willingness and readiness of people to take voluntary action. . . . A central question of public health has become: Why do people behave as they do?[1]

There can be little question that the successful conduct of many public health programs today requires both individual and community support. The public must be induced to participate in mass detection and immunization programs, to utilize available public health clinics, to support public health budgets and legislation, to change eating, drinking, and smoking habits, and to cooperate with local health units in dozens of different ways. The prevention, detection, and treatment of illness call for the full application of existing social science knowledge in such areas as community organization, communication, decision-making, and collective behavior. An understanding of the social and psychological factors that affect public and individual information, attitudes, and behavior regarding health programs or health measures is necessary if these programs are to be successful. It is axiomatic in public health that a poliomyelitis vaccine is ineffective unless people are immunized.

It may be briefly noted that not all sociological theories, concepts, and techniques are of equal importance, and perhaps more to the point, the significance they hold for social science may be quite different from their utility for public health. The importance of a concept for social science is related to a "pure" knowledge function, that is, the ordering of a great many different facts, while its importance for public health is greatly affected by the feasibility, efficiency, and cost with which it can be controlled. Thus some of the most brilliant sociological formulations have, as yet, little practicality for public health, while some of the most pedestrian results of social research in public health are received with great enthusiasm, often to the surprise of the sociologist. For example, in a mass tuberculosis screening study, the highly significant sociological finding that a large metropolitan neighborhood was virtually lacking in any formal community structure did not arouse nearly so much interest among public health practitioners as the finding that a successful way of getting people into a chest x-ray unit involved the use of music and "shills" or decoys.[2] The most pressing need in public health is for middle-range sociological theories that have high predictive value for social change and good administrative utility for producing or controlling such change.

In general, the public, especially that segment of it lowest in social, personal, and financial resources and yet highest in its need for health programs, is more noted for its ignorance, apathy, and resistance than for its knowledge, interest, and cooperation in regard to public health programs—or, for that matter, almost all forms of health and medical care. Only rarely can the consumer of potential public health services be approached on a purely rational basis. For most people, and in relation to most health programs, the rewards for participation are likely to be unrealistic and remote. Prevention does not have the same meaning and urgency as treatment of a painful or frightening illness.

This is especially true for the lower-income, slum areas where many of the major public health problems of today exist. This segment of the population has many more immediate and real problems than those offered by the prevention of some distant and unknown disease, or, even less salient, the lengthening of a life span by five or ten years. The narrow health horizons of this crucial group of the population makes them an extremely difficult target for public health activities. In the days of the communicable, infectious disease, it was often possible to circumvent the need for voluntary cooperation on the part of the individual through environmental or disease agent control measures on a communitywide basis, or through compulsory legislation to meet an obvious threat to the health of the public. Today, however, there is little that can be done to attack the chronic diseases or behavioral disorders paramount in the current health picture without the support and cooperation of the community. Individual responsibility is the keynote of modern preventive medicine; and a major goal of public health must be the determination of ways and means of either circumventing the need for individual action or of motivating the individual to cooperate in a voluntary program.

In a very real sense, public health must be marketed or sold to the health consumer. It is this marketing aspect of public health that provides the greatest challenge to applied sociology in the field of public health practice. And yet many social scientists shy away from this type of applied research, the reason probably being that the approach of many public health practitioners to the public has been in terms of merchandising a particular product. Certainly the "know-how" of the marketing professional is essential to the conduct of many current public health programs, but the appeal to and contribution of sociologists probably should be of a broader nature, involving an understanding of both sides of the "health equation"—public health and society. This attempt to align more successfully the nature, organization, distribution, and functioning of public health resources and services with the health needs, knowledge, perceptions, and behavioral patterns of the public can provide a real test for existing sociological knowledge concerning factors that influence social change and human behavior.

Somers and Somers in an excellent chapter on "Technological Change and Institutional Response" analyze the major difficulties faced by modern-day medical care. The main problem, as they see it, does not lie in the lack of medical knowledge or progress in the conquest of disease, but in the need to reorganize the societal arrangements for the provision of medical care. Resistance to such medical care innovation springs from "habit, tradition, self-interest, and the relative inflexibility of human institutions."[3]

The remainder of this chapter will examine some of these social barriers to the application of public health knowledge and techniques in terms of both community structure and individual behavior. In a general way, we may classify the types of problems involved in the conduct of public health programs according to two axes: (A) the emphasis upon individual behavior or community forces, and (B) the distinction between a single action or a continuing action. This is obviously an artificial separation since the individual cannot really be divorced from the community, while the community, in turn, is made up of individuals. However, if we view this framework as indicative of the major population target and time-orientation of a public health program, we can validly distinguish four broad areas of public health activity:

	Target Population	
	Community	Individual
Time-Orientation	Support	Behavior
Single action	A	C
Continued action	B	D

Each of these four cells presents a somewhat different problem in terms of a public health approach based on sociological principles. In the present discussion we can only characterize these briefly. Type A refers to those health programs that require only a single decision or action on the part of the community to make them effective, for example, fluoridation or the building of a health clinic. Type B requires not only the community decision to initiate a health activity but also continuing support of the activity over a longer period of time, for example, a neighborhood health council or home care program. Type C concerns those health programs that require just a single act on the part of the individual, for example, immunization or screening campaigns of a one-shot nature. Finally, Type D involves participation in health programs or the utilization of health facilities on a continuing basis, for example, child health stations or periodic chest x-rays.

The difficulty of securing the desired health action on an effective scale usually increases as we move from single action programs to programs requiring repeated action and from community programs to individual behavior. Thus public health seems to be most successful with programs that require a single marshaling of community support and least successful with those that depend upon the continued cooperation of separate individuals. As our discussion later will indicate, this analysis suggests that, whenever possible, a public health program should be developed in terms of a series of short-range actions aimed at long-range objectives and formulated in such a way that the community or group rather than the individual assumes responsibility for the decision and carrying out of the health activity.

Community Support and Action

An area of longstanding common interest to sociologists and public health workers is that of community factors influencing health action. Many of the first community studies in sociology were concerned with public health; in fact, some public health historians trace the beginning of the public health movement to community surveys by nonmedical men. Community studies on sanitary conditions by Chadwick in England and Shattuck in the United States in the early nineteenth century still stand as excellent examples of community research and have been credited with playing a major role in the development of the field of public health.

The community has traditionally been viewed as the main target of public health programs; in fact, public health has been called community medicine to distinguish it from private or clinical medicine. To be sure, all public health programs are conducted within a general community or public service framework but, for our purpose, we will limit the present discussion to those aspects of public health that deal specifically with community support of public health programs and community organization of health services.

It is becoming increasingly difficult to delimit the boundaries of the modern community. Urbanization has produced large cities in which all evidence of local communities has practically vanished. However, for the purposes of this analysis, we may take as our model the small local community with its formal and informal leadership structure, its local sources and distribution of power, its particular health needs and resources, and its own system of organization of health services. Our major problem will be to indicate the importance of social factors in determining the success or failure of health action programs in such a community. This aspect of public health has been approached by some sociologists as a problem in community decision-making processes.

Community factors in public health have occupied an especially large part of the attention of public health workers concerned with introducing new health measures into "underdeveloped" areas. A series of case studies by sociologists and anthropologists dealing with various attempts to change community health practices have produced overwhelming evidence to support the proposition that successful innovation must take into account existing community organization and local customs and values, and should involve local authority in the decision-making process.[4] An excellent review of sociocultural factors in intercultural health programs is given by Foster, who differentiates between cultural and social problems in community health action. The former concern the value system of the community and the emotional meaning of illness, as discussed in the previous chapter, while the latter are more related to problems of community structure and function. Foster lists eleven specific "cultural barriers" to change and seven "motivations" having a positive influence upon desired community health action. For example, he discusses the problem of "factionalism" resulting from disagreement among groups with opposing ideas and attitudes concerning the health program, and "communication" problems in translating health program objectives so that they are understood by the community. The suggestions he offers for research can serve as a valuable antidote to some of the more narrow emphases upon marketing "gimmicks."[5]

A penetrating analysis of community forces that need to be taken into account in attempting to introduce new social forms into "developing" areas is offered by Goodenough in a framework that brings together theory and empirical knowledge.[6]

Three major community health action studies have been conducted under the sponsorship of the Health Information Foundation in North Carolina,[7] Massachusetts,[8] and Michigan.[9] These studies have stressed the importance of the social organization and leadership structure of the community in determining community decisions regarding public health programs. Sanders offers a highly critical evaluation of these and other community action studies in terms of their oversimplification of such basic community processes as power structure, leadership, and decision-making. He is especially concerned with the fallacy in assuming that a "power clique" has free-floating power instead of influence in only the prescribed area of its own authority. He develops a paradigm for the analysis of community power in relation to the health system in terms of four dimensions: (a) type of leader, that is, organizational, functionaries; (b) systems involved—number of major systems, formal associations; (c) range of activities—specific, diffuse; and (d) duration of power—determinate, indeterminate. He then analyzes each of the major community health studies in terms of its specific contribution to this framework. He concludes with a series of ten propositions relating the community power structure and types of leadership to health action.[10]

A highly significant study of community organizational factors in a mass x-ray survey in New York City raises some disturbing questions concerning the relative low level of social organization in large urban areas. This study attributes the failure of determined efforts at securing community support for the mass x-ray program to the low social cohesion and ineffective community organization of large metropolitan neighborhoods. When there is no effective community organization to begin with, individual mobilization is a more apt description of what is needed than community organization. This study furthermore found that participation in the public health program was not attributable to high individual motivation and that nonparticipation was not the result of high resistance. In this type of health activity which carries little real meaning or salience for the individual, convenience, visibility, and activity seem more effective in producing the low-grade motivation needed for participation than complicated efforts at community organization.[11] This result will have great significance for our future discussion of individual behavior.

Perhaps the most extensively studied public health issue involving community organization and support is that of fluoridation. Several studies have been made and are currently in the field dealing with this important public health problem. The results of these research projects have demonstrated the effectiveness of community opposition to a public health measure despite the endorsement of all professional public health, medical, and dental associations. In general, these studies have shown that appeals for public support through a referendum are not an effective way of introducing fluoridation (the majority of such referenda are defeated); that the direct intervention of federal and state officials has not proved helpful; and that the issue has largely shifted from one of medical protection to a violation of the rights of individuals. A recent issue of the *Journal of Social Issues* summarizes a number of such community studies on fluoridation and analyzes the motivational factors of the opponents and proponents, the alignment of power within the community, and the relative effectiveness of various approaches toward instituting fluoridation. As noted by Paul, fluoridation offers an excellent opportunity for social research on community action.[12]

Community Opinion Processes. The issue of fluoridation quite dramatically illustrates the importance of an understanding of the social processes underlying public opinion. There is reason to believe that approaching public health action from the point of view of the concepts and principles of collective behavior will tell us why public health programs fail or succeed. The field of collective behavior attempts to understand such mass phenomena as social movements, public opinion, panic, and mob behavior. It concerns itself with those forces involved in the manipulation of public opinion such as propaganda, the mass media of communication, and pressure or special interest groups. As one State Commissioner of Health observed, "Public health is what the public wants." And what the public wants is in part the result of the public opinion process.

The conduct of public health programs requires a great deal of knowledge about the forces affecting and changing public opinion. The principles of communication and propaganda govern much of the work of public health educators. Changing the public's health habits—for example, those pertaining to diet, smoking, exercise—requires the highly skilled use of propaganda techniques and an understanding of the process of communication, both the formal mass media and the informal personal type.

Communication is a highly complex social process involving an awareness of such factors as the "two-step process" of public communication from mass media to opinion leader to general public, and the need to recognize the social context within which the communication takes place. Much of public communication takes place through a series of opinion leaders who have taken on, or been informally appointed to, the position of go-between. In all groups and in all communities, we find certain individuals who look, listen, and pass on information and ideas to other members of the group. These individuals occupy chief "gatekeeper" positions, and they are the people whose eyes and ears act as censors for the rest of the community. The Cornell Medical College program for introducing health innovations among the Navajo made deliberate and successful use of this principle by creating a role of a native "health visitor," to act as a communication link between the public health workers and the Navajo Indian.

There are many examples in public health of the need to approach the general public indirectly through some respected and accepted intermediary. Studies of successful and unsuccessful efforts at securing public support for fluoridation have indicated the greater wisdom of working through community leaders and enlisting the support of strategic individuals rather than attempting by public health education to obtain the approval of the public as a whole. We find that personal influence has a greater effect upon mothers' behavior in regard to poliomyelitis inoculations than do the formal media of communication. The formal media serve an important function in supplying these opinion leaders with information and arguments to be used in influencing the bulk of the public, but only rarely do these mass media appear to be effective in and of themselves.

In evaluating the influence of public health education on public opinion and behavior, it is important to recognize that this work is often done against the stream of powerful opposing countercommunications from private industry and special interest groups. Thus public health educators must attempt to infiltrate proper dietary habits in the face of private industry's promotion of candy and soft drinks; to counter the smoking habit while advertising budgets to sell cigarettes are infinitely larger than their own; to give advice on the use of drugs, cosmetics, and vitamins in opposition to a vast drug and vitamin industry. These examples underscore the need to view public health attempts at influencing the public's health habits within the context of all social forces affecting public opinion and behavior in the health area.

While current public opinion studies provide valuable information on the public's level of knowledge, attitudes, and behavior regarding various diseases and health services, a great deal remains to be done on the study of collective behavior in the field of public health. For example, we know very little about the way in which health fads develop, or the causes and effects of public panic in the face of epidemic scares, or the influence of various professional and trade associations, both in and out of the health field, upon public health legislation. We know practically nothing about the public's perception of public health problems or of the work of public health agencies. We need to know a lot more about public apathy, misinformation, and prejudice in regard to health and illness.

In the competition of health services with other public services such as education and welfare for the increasingly scarce tax dollar, the importance of understanding public demand for and support of public health programs cannot be overestimated. Social research can make an important contribution to public health by the examination of public apathy, disinterest, misinformation concerning and misunderstanding of public health programs, and by indicating ways and means of overcoming these obstacles to adequate health care.

A brief word should be said about the need to see community organization for health services and community decisions regarding health programs as an integral part of larger community services and decisions. Community action in the field of health cannot be divorced from social action in other community problem areas. As Koos has stated:

> . . . Community organization for health is in no sense an activity divorced from other forms of activity for community welfare . . . all community organization is interwoven in a common effort. Health, says modern research, is not to be found apart from a general welfare of the individual and the community. It consists not only of an absence of disease but also of a sense of general well-being, of adjustment to all of the forces that make up the intricacies of the society in which we live.[13]

Community Group Memberships. The community may be divided in a number of different ways into subgroups, each of which may be thought of as having its own particular organization and function, as being composed of members with somewhat different characteristics, and as having developed varying sets of attitudes and values. There is really no such thing as a single public. This basic fact of social structure has been implicitly recognized by the field of public health in its reporting of morbidity and mortality statistics according to demographic groups, and in its epidemiological approach to disease in terms of the differentiation of illness according to population groups.

The effect of group membership upon public health programs has been studied in regard to the lower utilization of health facilities by minority groups, the lower rate of polio inoculation among lower-income families, and the generally poorer participation of these lower social classes in mass detection programs. The public health approach to these socially deprived subgroups of the population cannot be based upon a middle-class public health philosophy; it must take into account the special problems of these various subcultural groups.

The provision of public health services to certain minority groups, such as the Negroes, Puerto Ricans, and Spanish-speaking Americans, is an especially important problem facing public health today. These groups show a much higher incidence of illness, and yet they are the most difficult to reach. The wide cultural barriers that keep these groups out of the mainstream of American life also cut them off from many available public health services.[14]

An interesting study has been made by Cornely and Bigman of the basic social factors that adversely affect the utilization of health services and knowledge concerning health among Negroes and whites of low-income status. As hypothesized by this project, in every urban community there are minority groups that are socially isolated and form a "hard core." This "hard core" all too often is resistant to change in attitudes and behavior in regard to health, disease, and medical care. The project has shown the importance of social group memberships in determining health status, health needs, utilization of preventive health services, eating and food patterns, knowledge of facilities and services, and general health values.[15] Comparable studies are much needed in the field of public health in order to plan public health programs that are geared to the health needs of these minority groups and that operate in accord with their values and behavioral patterns. A serious question may be raised as to whether it is these minority groups who are "disinterested and uninformed" about health services, or whether it is the public health worker who is "disinterested and uninformed" about the needs and cultural patterns of these groups.

Community Health Surveys. More on a fact-finding level, but with increasing attention to community structure and function, a large proportion of social research in the field of public health has been devoted to community health surveys aimed at determining the health needs and resources of a community, the current patterns of utilization of health facilities and services, information and attitudes toward disease and public health programs, and social and psychological factors affecting health behavior. Most major public health departments and many voluntary health agencies have at some time conducted community studies to evaluate the state of public knowledge, attitudes, and behavior in regard to their programs. As might be expected, these surveys have shown great variation in health needs, resources, information, attitudes, and behavior according to demographic and social group characteristics.

Two of the most comprehensive of these community studies were conducted by Koos in the United States[16] and by Spence and associates in England.[17] These studies conducted in different countries have documented the relevance of community attitudes and values for the conduct of public health programs. Other community studies have been made in relation to specific public health problems, such as Leighton and associates in Canada[18] and Srole and associates in New York in regard to mental disorder.[19] In fact, most current social research studies on disease and health programs include an analysis of community factors as essential information for understanding the nature of the problem.

A promising development in the field of public health relates to the establishment of community population laboratories in various schools of public health and health departments. These community laboratories are very similar to the community laboratories we find attached to several departments of sociology in universities, for example, the Detroit Area Study of The University of Michigan. The idea of such community population laboratories is to set up a single community area for concentrated research study. By studying the same area a great deal of information will accumulate on various aspects of community structure, leadership, disease patterns, health resources, and needs.

Individual Participation and Utilization

Community factors set the stage upon which the individual actor performs his daily tasks. The more highly structured the stage and the more prescribed the role of the actor, the more subject the individual will be to social constraints upon his behavior. However, within any given social structure, there is some room for individual freedom of choice and decision-making. Therefore, to understand and influence health action, the public health worker must take into account individual as well as community factors.

This need to deal with the individual health actor, as well as the community as a whole, has become increasingly important as public health has moved away from communicable disease control toward the preventive, therapeutic, and rehabilitative aspects of the chronic diseases and behavioral disorders. In the present-day health picture, greater reliance must be placed upon the individual's voluntary decision to participate in public health programs and to utilize available public health services. In the early days of public health, the communicable diseases could be attacked through authoritative control of environmental conditions, compulsory immunization, and forced isolation of diseased individuals. Today the focus is upon the chronic diseases, with prevention largely a matter of voluntary behavior involving basic changes in health habits and individual responsibility for early detection, combined with cooperation in long-term treatment and rehabilitation programs. Furthermore, the initial emphasis of the public health movement upon the building and provision of health facilities and services has shifted toward securing the utilization of such services by the public—again a matter of individual participation. It is quite apparent that public health has now entered an era of individual responsibility and voluntary cooperation which requires an understanding of the principles governing individual behavior.

We are now dealing with an area of primary concern to psychologists—the bases for individual behavior as compared to community action. Since this chapter is aimed primarily at an analysis of sociological contributions to public health, we will not devote much space to such psychological concepts as personality or motivation. In our opinion, however, it is inherently impossible to separate the social from the psychological factors in explaining human behavior. Both are involved. This is especially the case when one is dealing with the real-life behavior of the individual as a member of society. The pragmatic question for the public health worker becomes not one of psychological versus sociological concepts, but rather the determination of the relative importance of *both*, under varying conditions, in regard to specific types of health programs conducted in particular communities at a certain time. We may assume that at all times, but with differing relevance, health action will be based upon the decision-making processes of the individual as influenced by both the psychological factors of personal experience, belief, personality, and motivation and the sociological factors of status position, role functioning, and reference group influences. In some cases, the health act will be predominantly based on personal considerations; in other cases, it will represent primarily the influence of social forces. If we tend to accentuate the latter, it will be because of our own background and because, after all, this report is focused upon sociological contributions to public health.

In analyzing individual behavior from a "sociological" point of view, major emphasis will be placed upon role and status factors, reference group influences, and social interaction. This approach represents an analysis of the way in which the factors of who we are (our roles), where we belong (our statuses), and whom we look to for our models of behavior (our referents) affect our health behavior. These factors combine to produce our self-image and our group identifications. They establish our norms and values, and form the basis of our belief as to what constitutes "acceptable, appropriate, and desirable" health behavior.

Participation in Public Health Programs. One of the major objectives of public health is to increase the number of individuals who take part in mass screening programs such as tuberculosis, cancer, and diabetes detection, and who cooperate with mass immunization drives such as poliomyelitis or influenza. These are actions the individual must decide to take for his own good, and the extent of voluntary cooperation is the key to a successful or unsuccessful public health program. As described by Hochbaum:

> With the growing emphasis in public health on prevention and early detection of disease, there is an increasing need to enlist the voluntary participation of the public in health programs. Without such cooperation, many programs are destined to failure or to reduced effectiveness. Although the public stands to gain most from the success of health programs, its willingness to participate has all too often been disappointing, in spite of well-organized attempts to arouse popular interest and to make participation easy.[20]

Most voluntary mass participation programs are noted more for their failures than for their successes. Very rarely do such programs achieve the goal set for them by optimistic public health workers. Partly, this is the result of unrealistic expectations of the degree to which the public may be counted upon to cooperate voluntarily with any official request—expectations that are perhaps conditioned by the aura of the early nonvoluntary public health drives against the communicable diseases—and, partly, this is the result of a failure to recognize certain fundamental facts about the influencing of human behavior.

Polgar refers to the "fallacy of the empty vessel," whereby public health workers proceed as if they were pouring their activities and appeals into an empty void instead of an existing "popular health culture" which is already brimming over with accepted health notions and habits.[21] Perhaps one of the most common mistakes of public health workers is to assume "rationality" on the part of the public—that is, rationality from the public health professional's point of view. Such thinking assumes that given the facts about a disease and provided with a measure for combating it, the public will proceed logically to take advantage of the proffered public health program. What this approach fails to take into account is the generally low effectiveness of information alone as a determinant of behavior. Literally hundreds of studies have documented the fact that knowledge is rarely a sufficient basis for action. Attempts to change human behavior by a presentation of the "facts" alone are notably ineffectual.

Three important processes seem to intervene between facts and behavior: perception, interpretation, and salience. People observe selectively, that is, out of the myriad of messages with which they are being constantly bombarded; they perceive only those for which they already have an initial "set." Perhaps the greatest number of health messages never even reach the attention threshold of the individual. The interpretation or "meaning" of any given fact which the individual does perceive will depend to a large degree upon his previous experiences and his current needs. Thus subjectivity rather than objectivity will characterize the reaction of most individuals to the facts about disease. Finally, health knowledge is not the same as health action. To affect behavior, the health information must have salience for the individual in terms of the rewards to be obtained from acting on the basis of the facts. For many, if not most, individuals, especially those with limited social horizons and immediate needs, the rewards of preventive health behavior are too remote to carry much weight. The negative consequences of not acting are not real and dire enough to arouse the energy required to do something out of the ordinary, such as taking part in a public health program.

These basic principles were found to control the health behavior of a cross-section of low-income Negroes and whites surveyed in Washington, D. C.[22] As concluded by this study:

> . . . Health is not of primary importance to these families. There are too many matters in their everyday lives which would appear to have greater significance.
>
> . . . The concept of the ways and means by which health may be maintained as viewed by these families does not include certain measures which are of primary importance, such as immunizations, early diagnosis and prompt treatment. . . . The concern here, it is seen, is with matters of the moment and not with those which are more remote, and for conditions which are certainly neither pressing nor evident.

... Knowledge concerning a health procedure or verbal acceptance of its importance does not necessarily beget action on the part of these families in obtaining it. As a corollary, lack of knowledge about a procedure does not result in lack of action.

The foregoing analysis is obviously oversimplified and is intended only to highlight the importance of social and psychological factors in the operation of public health programs. We may characterize the difficulty of the problem for public health in terms of two major axes: (A) the degree of "meaning" the desired health action has for the individual, that is, his recognition of the disease as a personal threat; and (B) the degree of "effort" the action requires in terms of personal decision-making and activity. As charted below, we may hypothesize that the difficulty of securing individual participation in a public health program will increase as one moves from Cell A to Cell D.

	Degree of Recognition of Threat	
Degree of Effort Required	High	Low
Low	A	C
High	B	D

Thus it would be least difficult to induce the individual to participate in a smallpox vaccination program during the height of a threatened epidemic, especially if convenient and free inoculation stations were provided, while it would be most difficult to secure his cooperation in a diabetes screening program that required a series of tests. This general combination of personal threat and effort required has been found by a number of studies to underlie the success or failure of many public health programs. In an analysis of participation in a poliomyelitis vaccination campaign, Rosenstock attributes the decision to participate to two broad classes of factors: (a) personal readiness factors, consisting of perceived susceptibility and seriousness (comparable to recognition of threat); and (b) situational factors, among which he stresses convenience (comparable to effort). In addition, Rosenstock discusses the role of social pressure, which we will analyze later as an external force influencing the perception of threat or effort required.[23]

In another study of an Asian influenza vaccination program, Rosenstock and his colleagues concluded that the failure of individuals to be vaccinated, despite the possibility of a community-wide epidemic, stemmed from "a belief on the part of the vast majority of respondents that neither they nor their families were susceptible to Asian influenza, and a belief that Asian influenza was not much more serious, if more serious at all, than usual respiratory illness."[24] This finding again accentuates the importance of personal threat in determining the salience of a health act for the individual.

In an evaluation of research in the field of population control, Berelson stresses the overwhelming importance of such "down to earth" considerations as "not too much bother" and "effectiveness." He predicts that very little progress will be made in instituting birth control measures in a society unless the means for such control are so simplified that they require a minimum of individual initiative and result in a minimum of failures. He points out that even though the individual may have highly favorable attitudes and positive motivation toward family planning, he or she will not undertake the type of disciplined behavior required by such population control measures as abstinence or withdrawal, rhythm, contraceptives, or pills.[25] This is an example of the most difficult type of public health program, since it involves Cell D of the chart presented previously—individual behavior for a continuous period of time.

Other studies which support this hypothesis were conducted by Metzner and Gurin in relation to participation in a mass chest x-ray survey for tuberculosis detection in New York, and by Johnson and associates in regard to a poliomyelitis vaccination campaign in Florida. The New York study is particularly pertinent to our discussion, since it illustrates the kind of public health program to be found in Cell C of the previous table. The failure of the program to attain its goal of 80 per cent saturation of the population was attributed to the low salience of tuberculosis to the individual, while the degree of success attained was almost completely attributable to the "immediacy and convenience" of participation.[26]

The Florida study is particularly relevant because of its concern with interpersonal influences upon the individual. Such influences relate to the "social pressure" variable mentioned previously as important in Rosenstock's study of a poliomyelitis vaccination campaign. Both studies found that participation was closely related to the perception of the individual that other people were participating and *that he himself was expected to join them.* As reported by the Florida study:

> Belief that one's friends had taken the new vaccine had a particularly strong association with the respondent's own vaccine status. These informal interpersonal factors, membership in social organizations, social class, and education were the variables found by this survey to be the most powerful predictors of vaccine acceptance and rejection.[27]

The Florida study formulates the proposition on the importance of personal influences quite clearly:

> The respondent's perceived friends are his reference group. The actions he believes they took become one basis for deciding what is "the way my kind of people are supposed to act." Thus, persons who believed their friends took the oral vaccine also believed that their friends would approve and praise them for taking the vaccine, too. Similarly, where the persons important to the respondent were believed to have refused the vaccine, the respondent had the psychological experience group support for his nonacceptance.[28]

The implications of this study for public health programs are very direct. These programs need to develop approaches to the public that touch directly upon their customary patterns of behavior and attempt to make the health action "acceptable, desirable, and appropriate." The resistant groups of the population at present do not seem to find any worthwhile benefit in many of the current health programs. They simply do not see these health programs as meeting any of their "real" needs. In some way, the presentation of the health program must be changed so that some reward can be indicated to the individual besides the prevention of a disease about which he has no concern. Perhaps the most promising redefinition is not in terms of "good" health behavior, but rather a change in the picture of how people like themselves *should* behave in regard to the public health programs. The same idea is emphasized in the Florida study's final recommendation for the conduct of public health programs.

The data of this study do not indicate the necessity of factual discussion of the dangers of polio or the merits of vaccine. All that appears necessary is for people to feel they have a group of friends and to believe that most or all of these friends will be taking or have taken vaccine. Fostering this collective perception should greatly increase vaccine acceptance.[29]

This approach to public health programs, which takes cognizance of the low salience of purely health appeals for the public and which stresses a kind of social conformity requiring greater motivation to resist than to comply, offers an interesting possibility for public health practice based on a sociological rather than a psychological approach. This notion underlies Hochbaum's statement in regard to participation in a tuberculosis screening program:

Even when this state of (psychological) readiness is absent or of very low intensity, people were found to come for x-rays *in response to external influences alone.* These may be influences exerted by other individuals or groups. In other words, people may come for x-rays not for any health-relevant reasons, but to please other people, to be accepted by their groups, and the like.[30]

The same basic idea of circumventing motivational appeals keyed to the threat of disease, where the perception of such a threat cannot be made real to the person, is expressed by Metzner and Gurin in their final conclusions.

Much in our society depends on building into it automatic, unavoidable acts which are not directly motivated toward the goals they achieve nor represent conscious decisions to be good or safe . . . and what success we have had in vaccination lies more in making it a part of the relationship with a pediatrician or the school system than in increasing appreciation of and desire for immunity.[31]

This, then, is one of the major contributions sociology can offer to public health practice—the development and testing of methods and techniques that make the desired health behavior part of the prevailing value system and pattern of behavior of the individual, based not upon appeals to his health but rather upon the appropriateness of the behavior itself. Thus mothers may be influenced to take their children to health stations for polio shots not so much in terms of protecting the child from disease as in terms of "what every 'good' mother is expected to do" and "what other mothers like me are doing." This suggestion is supported by the findings of the Washington, D. C., study of the health behavior of low-income families:

> . . . It may not be necessary for people to be informed provided they can be motivated by other means. The mothers who took their children to be vaccinated, although ignorant about the disease, may have been motivated by the thought that this is what is expected of good mothers.[32]

The mother's definition of such action as appropriate to her role as a mother rather than simply advantageous to the health of the child was also found to be highly significant by Clausen and associates in their study of participation in the poliomyelitis vaccine trials.[33]

Public health professionals have long known that a public health program that did not depend upon individual initiative and effort but upon professional action would be more likely to be effective. The approach being proposed here is the removal of certain health acts from the area of individual decision-making by making them, wherever possible, a part of the socially accepted way of behaving. This is not to say that such programs will be easy to carry out, only that they will offer a new line of attack more congruent with the demands of current public health needs. Additional support for this sociological approach is given by Simmel and Ast, who emphasize the greater relevance of social categories as opposed to psychological classifications for public health action.

> But public health cannot attempt to influence the public one by one, psyche by psyche. However fascinating they may be, psychological phenomena are only of secondary interest to us. A psychological classification of people is of little use if we cannot locate the different psychological types in the community. The constancies which are likely to be useful in the design and focusing of health education programs and strategies are those whose occurrence or nonoccurrence, in any case whose relative frequencies of occurrence distinguish between categories of people initially defined in social or ecological terms.[34]

In proposing this particularly sociological approach to the conduct of public health programs, a brief word should be said about the testing of sociological concepts in the crucible of real-life experiences. In its present stage of development, sociology is a long way from being able to offer to public health a truly applied "social engineering." This is obvious from the fragmented, disorganized, nonadditive nature of current applied research in sociology. At this stage of early growth, it is premature to judge the validity of sociological concepts and theories in terms of their practical utility or "correctness" in solving an applied problem.

To the public health practitioner, and at times even to the sociologist working on a public health problem, the extent to which sociological concepts hold up "under fire" assumes exaggerated importance. For example, while sociology may have an excellent theoretical formulation of social class pressures that interfere with mass screening programs or community forces that resist fluoridation, the task of the practicing professional is to turn this knowledge to his advantage. Unless he is shown how he can use such knowledge to motivate Mr. A. to appear for a chest x-ray or Community Y to vote favorably on a fluoridation referendum, he is likely to feel that the knowledge is invalid. Unsuccessful manipulation is not a test of the scientific worth of a concept—even though it may lead the public health practitioner to conclude that social science has little practical utility for him.

Many of the problems public health is facing today are not amenable to manipulation, even granted that social science can determine why they exist. Mass ignorance, apathy, and resistance are not easily overcome. And yet, too often, the public health practitioner will turn over some of his toughest problems to the social scientist and, because the problem is one involving social change, expect the social scientist to tell him not what the problem is or why it exists, but what he can do (often immediately and without too much effort) to correct it. Perhaps a lesson from medical research is in order. The fact that medical research to date has not found the cures for the major killers of modern society—cardiovascular disease and cancer—is no reason for labeling such research useless.[35] Some of the same kind of tolerance is necessary and appropriate for social science research in the public health field.

The Epidemiological Model and Health Action

It may be helpful to the public health worker striving to understand the significance of social science principles to translate one of the common social science models for explaining behavior into epidemiological terms.[36] This comparison not only may clarify the common meeting ground of public health and sociology, and thus increase mutual understanding and communication; it should also provide insight into why current trends in disease and medical care are moving public health and sociology inexorably closer together.

As originally developed by Lazarsfeld, one classification scheme for analyzing action by the individual consists in the separation of three types of factors: (1) the internal *tendencies* of the individual that predispose him toward or away from the observed behavior; (2) the external *influences* in the environment that favor or oppose the course of action; and (3) the inherent *attributes* of the action itself or the object or goal of the action that make it attractive or unattractive to the individual. This is a highly oversimplified statement of the intimate interrelationships between these three sets of factors, but for the sake of this comparison, we need not be concerned with the complexities of the model.

There is an enlightening parallel between this threefold classification and the classical trilogy of epidemiological analysis. In epidemiology we also view the causes of disease in terms of three major groups of factors: (1) the *host* factors, which include all those characteristics present in the human individual that increase or decrease his chances of contracting the disease; (2) the *environmental* factors, which surround the individual and which deter or aid the development of the disease; and (3) the *agent* factors present in the disease-causing object or process itself, which determine its ability to produce the disease state. There is a direct parallel, which is more than a coincidental analogy, between internal tendencies and the host, external influences and the environment, and inherent attributes and the agent.

The significance of this parallel has important implications both for understanding the etiology and prevention of disease and for the explanation and change of human behavior. In both cases we seek, first, to discover what characteristics of the individual are related to either the disease process or the course of action. In the case of disease, these are likely to be biological or physiological states, while in human behavior, they are more likely to refer to the psychological and social characteristics of the individual. Thus it is not difficult to understand why, when the disease itself becomes psychosomatic or a behavioral disorder or a chronic condition closely allied to the individual's way of living, we have the growth of "social" epidemiology concerned with the incidence and prevalence of disease according to the group memberships and psychological characteristics of the individual. Secondly, we look at the environment; for disease states, we seek to determine which factors in the environment produce or enhance the etiological process, while for human behavior, we attempt to determine the effect of outside influences upon individual action. Again, we note a shift in current epidemiology from concentration upon the physical environment to increasing concern with the social environment. Finally, we study the agent itself to determine, in the case of disease, which agent is carrying the disease and how this agent infects the host and, in the case of human behavior, what characteristics of the action or the objective of the action lead the individual to seek or avoid the necessary behavior to attain the objective. When, as is often true in the chronic diseases or behavioral disorders, there is no specific infectious agent involved, the social and individual objectives that underlie the way of life of the individual become basic "agents" in the etiology of disease.

We conclude this brief analogy by examining the implications of the aforementioned similarities between social science and epidemiology for public health action. The primary objective of public health is the prevention of disease. As we have seen, such prevention has traditionally been concerned with the elimination of conditions in the physical environment conducive to disease, such as sanitation, and the neutralizing of the infectious agent either by decreasing its potency or building up the resistance of the host. Today we may view the goals and means of public health in a similar way, only accenting a *change in human behavior* as a necessary intermediate objective in the prevention of disease. Retaining the same basic concepts of classical epidemiology, we seek to change human behavior in order to (1) decrease the *exposure* of the host to disease-causing ways of life, such as smoking, drinking, or stress, and the *susceptibility* of the host to the inevitable challenges to health in modern living; (2) increase the *supportive* forces in the social environment of the individual both to help him avoid unhealthy acts and to take advantage of health-inducing measures; and (3) decrease the *effectiveness* or virulence of the disease-causing processes themselves so that exposure is to some degree nullified. In other words, the focus of combating disease is still upon the host, the agent, and the environment; only the goal has shifted from the end disease state itself to the intervening human behavior. When the human behavior itself becomes the disease, as in the case of some behavioral disorders, then we need not even posit behavior as an intervening variable. And it is in the development of the new methods necessary for achieving this intermediate goal of changed human behavior that sociology has its greatest contribution to make to public health practice.

NOTES TO CHAPTER V

1. Editorial, *American Journal of Public Health*, vol. 49, April, 1959, p. 536.
2. Metzner, Charles A., and Gerald Gurin, *Personal Response and Social Organization in a Health Campaign*. University of Michigan, Bureau of Public Health Economics, Research Series No. 9, Ann Arbor, 1960.
3. Somers, Herman M., and Anne R. Somers, *Doctors, Patients, and Health Insurance*. Brookings Institution, Washington, 1961, p. 458.
4. Paul, Benjamin D., editor, *Health, Culture, and Community*. Russell Sage Foundation, New York, 1955.
5. Foster, George M., *Problems in Intercultural Health Programs*. Social Science Research Council, Pamphlet 12, New York, 1958.
6. Goodenough, Ward H., *Cooperation in Change:* An Anthropological Approach to Community Development. Russell Sage Foundation, New York, 1963.
7. Kimball, Solon T., and Marion Pearsall, *The Talledga Story:* A Study in Community Process. University of Alabama Press, Tuscaloosa, Ala., 1954.
8. Hunter, Floyd, R. C. Schaffer, and C. G. Sheps, *Community Organization:* Action and Inaction. University of North Carolina Press, Chapel Hill, 1956.
9. Sower, Christopher, *Community Involvement*. The Free Press, Glencoe, Ill., 1957.
10. Sanders, Irwin T., "Public Health in the Community" in Freeman, Howard, Sol Levine, and Leo G. Reeder, editors, *Handbook of Medical Sociology*. Prentice-Hall, Inc., Englewood Cliffs, N. J., 1963, pp. 369–396.

11. Metzner, Charles A., and Gerald Gurin, *op. cit.*
12. Paul, Benjamin D., "Fluoridation and the Social Scientist: A Review," *Journal of Social Issues*, vol. 17, 1961, p. 7. This entire issue is devoted to fluoridation research.
13. Koos, Earl L., "New Concepts in Community Organization for Health," *American Journal of Public Health*, vol. 43, April, 1953, pp. 468–469.
14. Suchman, Edward A., and Lois S. Alksne, "Communicating Across Cultural Barriers," *American Catholic Sociological Review*, vol. 22, Winter, 1961, pp. 306–313.
15. Cornely, Paul B., and Stanley K. Bigman, *Cultural Considerations in Changing Health Attitudes*. Howard University, Washington, D. C., December, 1961. Mimeographed.
16. Koos, Earl L., *The Health of Regionville*. Columbia University Press, New York, 1954.
17. Spence, James C., and others, *A Thousand Families in Newcastle Upon Tyne*. Oxford University Press, London, 1954.
18. Leighton, Alexander, *My Name Is Legion*. Basic Books, Inc., New York, 1959. See also Hughes, Charles, and others, *Cove and Woodlot*, Basic Books, Inc., New York, 1960.
19. Srole, Leo, and others, *Mental Health in the Metropolis*. McGraw-Hill Book Co., New York, 1962.
20. Hochbaum, Godfrey M., *Public Participation in Medical Screening Programs*. U.S. Public Health Service, Publication No. 572, Government Printing Office, Washington, 1958, p. 1.
21. Polgar, Steven, "Health and Human Behavior: Areas of Interest Common to the Social and Medical Sciences," *Current Anthropology*, vol. 3, April, 1962, pp. 159–205. This review presents an extensive bibliography of the literature.
22. Cornely, Paul B., and Stanley K. Bigman, *op. cit.*, pp. 168–169.
23. Rosenstock, Irwin M., and others, "Why People Fail to Seek Poliomyelitis Vaccination," *Public Health Reports*, vol. 74, February, 1959, pp. 98–104.
24. Rosenstock, Irwin, and others, *The Impact of Asian Influenza on Community Life*. U.S. Public Health Service, Publication No. 766, Government Printing Office, Washington, 1960, p. 75.
25. Berelson, Bernard, "Communication, Communication Research, and Family Planning," *The Emerging Techniques in Population Research*, Proceedings of the 39th Conference of the Milbank Memorial Fund, New York, 1963.
26. Metzner, Charles A., and Gerald Gurin, *op. cit.*
27. Johnson, A. L., and others, *Epidemiology of Polio Vaccine Acceptance*. Florida State Board of Health, Monograph No. 3, 1962, p. 98.
28. *Ibid.*, p. 42.
29. *Ibid.*, pp. 90–91.
30. Hochbaum, Godfrey M., *op. cit.*, p. 21.
31. Metzner, Charles A., and Gerald Gurin, *op. cit.*, p. 33.
32. Cornely, Paul B., and Stanley K. Bigman, *op. cit.*, p. 169.
33. Clausen, John A., Morton A. Seidenfeld, and Leila C. Deasy, "Parent Attitudes Toward Participation of Their Children in Polio Vaccine Trials," *American Journal of Public Health*, vol. 44, December, 1954, pp. 1526–1536.
34. Simmel, Arnold, and David B. Ast, "Some Correlates of Opinion on Fluoridation," *American Journal of Public Health*, vol. 52, August, 1962, p. 1269.
35. As James points out, "Of the 19 leading causes of death in New York City, only 2 represent conditions which can be controlled effectively by existing health programs." James, George, "Community Disease Detection Programs," *New York State Journal of Medicine*, vol. 61, August 15, 1961, p. 2757.
36. This translation, in reverse, should, of course, prove helpful to the social scientist in understanding one of the basic explanatory models in public health for the occurrence of disease. We state it in the present form in order to accent the contribution that social science concepts can make to public health.

VI

ORGANIZATIONAL AND OCCUPATIONAL STRUCTURE OF PUBLIC HEALTH

PUBLIC HEALTH constitutes one of the major social subsystems of a community. As such, it displays the significant features of any social system: (1) an organizational structure including administrative arrangements for the provision of health services; (2) a circumscribed set of functions defining its goals and objectives; (3) a group of functionaries to carry on its activities; (4) a rationale or ideology that justifies its existence; (5) a set of tools and techniques for performing its functions; and (6) an interrelationship with other systems in the community, such as education and welfare. The analysis and interpretation of these basic social characteristics of public health comprises a major area of sociological investigation which may be labeled the "sociology of public health." As defined by Straus in relation to the sociology of medicine, this area is "concerned with studying such factors as the organizational structure, role relationships, value system, rituals, and functions of medicine as a system of behavior."[1] This approach to health as a social system has been developed in some detail by Sanders in terms of community factors related to public health.[2]

As in the case of the previous applications of sociology to public health problems, an organizational and occupational analysis of the field of public health has both basic significance and applied utility. Knowledge concerning the structure, operation, goals, values, and personnel of the health field increases our understanding of an essential component of the total social system. The study of public health organizations can provide basic data on the structure and function of social organizations in general, for, as Foster has observed:

> A public health organization . . . can be looked upon as a society with a specific culture. . . . It is composed of persons of both sexes, of different ages, organized in a hierarchy marked by power and authority, with well-defined roles and occupational specialization, with mutually recognized rights and obligations. This society shares common values, it engages in professional rituals, and it operates on assumptions that normally are not questioned. The cohesive and divisive forces within it, the stresses and strains, and the unifying elements are similar to those found in other societies.[8]

Research on organizational and occupational factors in public health also has immediate practical application to problems in public health administration and to the recruitment and training of public health personnel. The growing complexity of public health services has created a serious need for the development of an administrative science of public health based upon tested principles of program planning and operation. The supervision of a modern public health agency, especially in a large metropolitan area, calls for an understanding of bureaucratic structure, staff organization, personnel policies, financial budgeting, and public relations, along with the many other skills of executive management. Very few public health officials have received formal training in public health administration, although the number is increasing rapidly as graduate schools of public health emphasize the administrative aspects of public health practice.

Similarly, the study of public health personnel can provide useful information for meeting current problems of personnel shortages. These shortages are particularly acute at the professional level of public health physicians, nurses, and engineers. Occupational sociology has a valuable contribution to make toward an understanding of the positive and negative factors that attract or repel prospective candidates and subsequently lead to job satisfaction or dissatisfaction. Research on the socialization process in graduate public health education and on the definition of occupational roles in public health practice can point up sources of strain and conflict between expectations and realizations. Personnel studies can examine such problems as working conditions, interpersonal relationships, communication, and leadership.

The present chapter will summarize and evaluate sociological contributions, first, to public health organizational problems and, second, to public health occupational problems. In general, very little social research has been done in these two areas despite their obvious importance. As yet, no systematic study has been made of the structure and function of a public health department, although a large number of evaluations have been made of specific service programs. Similarly, no detailed studies have been made of graduate training in schools of public health comparable to those made of medical students.

Structural-Functional Analysis of Public Health Organizations

The general nature of public health organization in the United States has already been described in Chapter III. We noted the complexity of the multitude of official and voluntary health agencies on the national, state, and local levels. According to a study made by the United States Public Health Service in 1950, separate agencies of the state government alone participating in some form of health activity at that time totaled 60 in number.[4] Even in regard to official health agencies, marked variability occurs among the states in the assignment of responsibility and in the operation of health programs.

Obviously, no single pattern of organization can encompass all of these differing agencies and activities. In general, we may group them into four main types, although these may overlap considerably: (1) official or public agencies, (2) voluntary or nonprofit agencies, (3) hospitals and nursing homes, and (4) health-related organizations. By far the greatest number of structural-functional analyses has been made of hospitals, especially mental hospitals. In an analysis of 90 social research projects concerned with social systems in the health field, Wellin and Seacat found that 90 per cent of all such studies dealt with hospitals, about equally divided between psychiatric and general hospitals. The major emphasis of these studies was upon social structure and role relationships.[5] Hospitals provide a natural setting for social research on organizational problems. They are highly complex structures with a wide variety of functions and personnel, and yet they constitute highly self-contained units in and of themselves. Hospital administration is a rapidly expanding field of professional activity, while the hospital "business" in the United States encompasses more than 7,000 hospitals, employing about 1,500,000 full-time workers and admitting approximately 25,000,000 patients each year.[6]

These organizational studies of hospitals are valuable to public health in highlighting the importance of administrative arrangements and staff interaction in the provision of health services. Burling, Lentz, and Wilson, in a study of six private, nonprofit hospitals, found that the strong differentiation of tasks in the health field creates serious problems of communication.[7] These communication problems become intensified by a dual system of authority, one professional and one administrative,[8] which creates many problems in staff interaction.[9] Organizational conflicts have been found to have a deleterious effect upon the quality of patient care.[10] Several interesting experiments have documented the fact that changing the lines of authority and communication can result in patient progress.

At the present time, we lack similar organizational studies of public health units, as Rosen and Wellin have pointed out in their comprehensive bibliography on the social sciences and public health.[11] McEwen, in an unpublished study, has analyzed the structure and function of a municipal health center in an attempt to determine the different types of work-orientations of persons occupying different positions in the health centers and to relate these to certain types of role relationships (power, status, communication) as well as to elements of public health ideology. The organizational problems of local health units are currently being studied by the Social Science Unit of the Harvard School of Public Health to ascertain what factors facilitate or impede cooperation among official and voluntary organizations offering health services to the community.

An analysis of the structure of local health units indicates that the prevailing organizational pattern of the local government influences the kind of health organization established. In general, there are four major classifications of the 1,577 official local health organizations: single county health units (58 per cent), local health districts (15 per cent), city health units (20 per cent), and state health districts (7 per cent). The most common form of organization is the local health district characterized by the consolidation of the resources of contiguous counties or other political subdivisions.[12] Such combined local units can offer more efficient and economical health services. Atwater describes this trend toward consolidation as follows:

> It was, of course, apparent more than a decade ago that we must have county or district health departments to deliver the essentials of modern public health and that the thousands of village, town, township, and city departments then existing were manifestly inadequate. To be sure, many of these inadequate departments still exist in spite of the march of consolidation and integration. But there is no longer any doubt of the need for larger administrative units.[13]

The effect of the pattern of local government upon the consolidation of health units can be seen in the geographical variations existing in the United States. The city, town, or municipality type of independent local health unit is found most frequently in the Northeast, whereas multi-county health units flourish in the Southeast and South Central portions of the country. One result of this variation is to decrease the proportion of the population that remains uncovered by the protection of full-time health services in the Southeast (8 per cent) as compared to the Northeast and North Central regions (43 per cent).[14]

In this report we cannot go into the diversity of organizational forms to be found in regard to specific health programs or services, or into the many organizational problems produced by the separation of public health, mental health, and medical welfare. Public health services have been referred to as "a many-splintered thing." Services tend to be fragmented and discontinuous and, with some justification, multi-problem families may more aptly be described as single families with multi-agency problems. Roemer and Wilson have documented the high degree of fractionation in organized health services even in a semirural county,[15] while a recent pilot study by Connery showed formidable fractionation and discontinuity of mental and other public health services in metropolitan areas.[16] As summarized by Donabedian and Axelrod:

It is apparent from the foregoing that a major characteristic of the organization of medical care in this country is its lack of organization. . . . Everywhere one is confronted with shortages, maldistribution, haphazard growth, and inefficient use of scarce and valuable resources. What is required is a broad, flexible, and carefully coordinated system in which appropriate services are readily available and continuously adapted to the patients' needs.[17]

The relationship of public health agencies to each other and to the community in general is an area of growing concern as the need for both interagency cooperation and community support of health programs becomes more imperative. Etzioni stresses the area of interorganizational relationships as particularly important to an analysis of organizational structure related to environment.[18] Johns and de Marche examine the barriers to interagency cooperation and list such factors as differences in professional philosophy, vested interests, lack of knowledge concerning agency objectives, and pressures of national organizations.[19] They propose a typology of interagency relationships based upon the degree of joint consultation, planning, and program operation. Levine and White attribute the need for cooperation between health agencies to the scarcity of human and nonhuman resources in the health field and call for an exchange of services.[20]

Conflict between health organizations usually arises when two agencies attempt to reach the public with the same type of health program. In the field of public health this competitive interest lies at the heart of many of the conflicts between official and voluntary health agencies and among the voluntary health agencies themselves. In the United States over 100,000 voluntary health and welfare agencies now receive more than $1.5 billion annually in public contributions. These agencies compete with one another for financial support and for predominance in their chosen field of activity. The result, as evaluated by Hamlin, is duplication and wastefulness, and the need is for greater public control and cooperative action.[21]

To this conflict among voluntary health agencies must be added an increasing competition of interests among public agencies in regard to public health, mental health, and medical welfare. In most instances, these three programs are operated by separate agencies. The separate development of these three fields has both disciplinary and governmental roots. Public health originated as a branch of medicine concerned with community preventive health; mental health sprang from clinical psychiatry with a strong emphasis upon therapy and the individual patient; while medical welfare arose as one aspect of social welfare and social work with its major focus upon family casework. Today all three are coming closer together as public health moves into the area of medical care, mental health into community psychiatry, and medical welfare into prevention, integrated care, and rehabilitation.

There can be little question that a great deal of research is needed on the problems of organizational structure and function in the field of medical care. In the future it is probable that official public health units will be called upon to perform an important integrative function in bringing together the various disparate health services in a community. Levine and White examined the qualifications of the public health physician for this role of community coordinator of health services and found him a likely candidate with his training in medicine, community organization, and program operation.[22] This is a role also assigned to the public health professional by Dixon, who sees him as "the public health generalist of the future" whose responsibility would be to coordinate the various community health services on some "broad-based technic of public health practice."[23]

Before this type of development can take place, a great deal more will have to be learned about the problems of public health organization and administration. Research is almost completely lacking on this important aspect of public health practice. What is known and taught today is largely a translation of the principles of business and public administration to public health administration. These include such standard problems as integration versus autonomy, centralization versus decentralization, scalar versus functional organizational structures, staff versus line organization of services and functions, and the general analysis of administrative management, including hierarchical levels and degrees of complexity, extra-departmental and intra-departmental administrative functions, fiscal operation and personnel management. To be sure, the modern public health officer must be acquainted with these general principles of administrative science, but what is seriously needed are specific studies of problems in public health administration. As pointed out by the National Health Advisory Council in 1961,"given the complexity of modern therapy, diligence and skill in administration are required to provide the trained personnel, facilities, finances, and other components necessary to provide the best possible medical care for the population served."[24]

A good analysis of the role of administrative science in the field of medical care is offered by Demerath, who lists seven foci for future research: (1) analysis of programs of medical care, (2) coordination and intraorganization impacts of programs or units on each other, (3) costs and financing of medical care, (4) studies of the health professions, (5) utilization of medical facilities and services, (6) innovations and innovative techniques in medical care administration, and (7) methodological studies.[25] Given the inevitably greater participation of public health organizations in medical care, the need for administrative research in the field of public health becomes of paramount importance.

Sociological studies of the structure and function of public health organizations can contribute a great deal toward the more effective operation of public health services. This is practically virgin territory for the exploration of such problems as role and status relationships within health departments, channels of communication and staff interaction, the distribution and exercise of power, and agency relationships with the community, with other health organizations, and with the various groups and individuals to whom it offers services. Research on such problems not only can provide answers to urgent administrative problems in public health, but also contribute significantly to the growing body of sociological knowledge on the functioning of large organizations in modern society.

Occupational Analysis of Public Health Field

The growth of public health as a professional field of activity in recent years has been both rapid and widespread. Expansion has taken place, however, in the face of immediate needs without too much time for speculation about the long-range nature of public health work or the formulation of clear-cut occupational categories with prescribed roles and statuses. For the most part, personnel have been transferred or borrowed from existing health fields, and the definition of job requirements, duties, and working relationships has been built up pragmatically over the years to meet existing demands. One result of this more or less haphazard growth has been the proliferation of many different occupational categories whose functions have been defined more in terms of traditional roles than in answer to particular public health needs. In many cases, public health work has been limited to a part-time activity on the part of medical personnel whose primary professional identification and allegiance has remained with their original field of training. This "borrowing" and part-time commitment has interfered with the growth of a clearly defined professional field of public health and has led to frequent misunderstandings and a lack of appreciation of public health work on the part of both traditional medicine and the lay public.

The need to overcome the public's misconception of public health work is supported by the findings of a study of a cross-section of low-income families in Washington, D. C. This study concluded:

> Of particular significance, however, is the image which those families have of the official health department. It is viewed as a curative rather than preventive service unit; it has been saddled with garbage disposal and sewage treatment; and the majority of the families are not aware of having used any of its services. This then means that the health department in a city such as this and for families represented here must put a lot of effort in order to reach into these areas and alter the image. Thus, the public may come to view the health department not as a symbol of authority or of pauperism, or as one synonymous with hospital or medical care, and thereby come to accept its services more readily.[26]

A similar conclusion is reached by Simmel and Ast following their analysis of community reactions to proposed fluoridation of the water supply.

> It is our impression that public health organizations, at any rate the vast majority of their activities, are almost invisible to the public.

> ... It would appear that one long-run implication for public health is to work toward generating a more favorable and more visible public image of itself.[27]

As the emphasis of public health work shifts toward preventive, therapeutic, and rehabilitative programs for the chronic diseases and behavioral disorders, public health as a health profession is bound to rise in prestige among both the medical profession and general public. Increasingly, public health programs will be staffed by full-fledged, full-time public health workers. To quote Howard Ennes, "Public health service is no part-time job—it requires full-time, trained, professional personnel dedicated to their work."[28]

This need for a distinctive occupational field of public health was anticipated in 1915 by Rosenau, who said:

> The time has long since gone by when the physician can spend a few hours from his busy day to look after the duties of the health office. The situation demands the entire time and energy of those who consecrate their lives to the public welfare. . . . Public health work is becoming, in fact, has already become, a separate profession. . . . Public health service, as a career, must be an end in itself. It is often difficult and sometimes impossible to bend the physician into a health officer. The ordinary medical training does not qualify a person to be a health officer.[29]

Progress in as professionally conservative a field as medicine comes slowly and today, almost fifty years after Rosenau's statement, physicians serving as part-time health officers and as part-time clinicians still outnumber full-time public health physicians by six to one—8,600 to 1,400 in 1960.[30] This does not include physicians in school health programs, most of whom also serve on a part-time basis. Public health as a career for physicians still continues to occupy relatively low status. As Baumgartner has pointed out:

> All too often the physician going into public health was either a disabled or disgruntled private practitioner. In many areas, selection of health officers at best consisted of a form of retirement for well-thought-of clinicians who had reached an age at which they were no longer able to carry on the rigorous needs of clinical practice. During

the past couple of decades, more and more physicians going into public health work have chosen that specialty on its merit.[31]

Part of the explanation for the current status of the public health occupations lies in the historical background of public health work. Public health as a professional field of activity is quite young. Full-time health departments actually came into existence only about the time that the first World War began, while it was not until 1916 that the first distinct school of public health was established at the University of Pennsylvania. This move was followed by the rapid growth of 45 schools granting 18 different kinds of degrees in public health by the year 1939.[32] This situation was remedied in 1941 by the establishment of an Association of Schools of Public Health and an accreditation system developed by the American Public Health Association. Today professional training in public health is fairly well established in 14 graduate schools of public health in the United States and Canada. As summarized by Troupin:

> It is obvious that schools of public health now occupy an established place in the national educational picture. Although they do not have the long years of background experience of schools of medicine, dentistry, nursing and others in the health field, schools of public health have made considerable progress in only a few decades of existence. As experience accumulates and as the institutions engage in more study and analysis of their own activities, even greater steps forward may be anticipated.[33]

Currently, an extensive exploration of schools of public health and professional education in the field of public health entitled "The Joint Committee Study of Education for Public Health" is being conducted by Shepard and Elling. This comprehensive study should greatly increase our understanding of professional education in the field of public health.[34]

A second difficulty in the growth of professional status of the public health worker arises from the wide variety of occupational groupings to be found in the field of public health. A United States Public Health Service survey of local health units in 1960 classified the 44,007 full-time employees of official health agencies into 23 different categories as follows:

Public health nurses	14,384
Clerks	9,878
Professional sanitarians	6,112
Other sanitation personnel	2,433
Maintenance and service	1,839
Laboratory personnel	1,489
Public health physicians	1,402
Clinic nurses	647
Administrative management	509
Engineers	446
Dental hygienists	395
Public health investigators	393
X-ray technicians	355
Public health dentists	309
Health educators	281
Veterinarians	245
Medical social workers	228
Analysts and statisticians	217
Psychiatric social workers	189
Physical therapists	158
Nutritionists	136
Psychologists	104
All others	1,858
Total	44,007

It is obvious from this census that the field of public health is composed of a heterogeneous mixture of medical, paramedical, and auxiliary personnel. The largest professional category by far is the public health nurse, followed by sanitarians, laboratory personnel, and physicians. This combination of professional and nonprofessional personnel, some of whom are educated in the medical sciences and others who are not, some of whom render medical services and others who have little to do directly with the individual client, undoubtedly creates a confused image of the public health worker, which tends to detract from his occupational prestige. In general, studies of the status hierarchy of health occupations place physicians and dentists at the top of the scale, nurses, laboratory technicians, health educators, and so on, in the middle range, and clerks and maintenance personnel at the bottom. Some of the major areas of occupational conflict in public health today spring from the jealously guarded "professional" status of the more medically trained groups, who fear a downgrading of their prestige should less qualified personnel be permitted to enter their ranks.

The field of public health offers a particularly challenging area for analysis and research to the occupational sociologist. The sociology of work has a distinct and highly significant contribution to make to current public health personnel problems. As yet, there have been no systematic studies of public health workers, although, as we shall see later, a number of studies have been made of the public health nurse and currently several research projects on the public health physician are in progress. There is a great need for research on occupational roles and role relationships within public health organizations, on social stratification and the hierarchy of authority within public health, on the division of labor and resultant status and prestige conflicts, on the channels of communication and influence, and on informal structure and organization.

A fair amount of social research has been conducted on the health professions other than public health.[35] We mention these studies briefly, together with the few that have been conducted in the field of public health, to indicate the type of problem that can be studied with benefit to the field of public health. These studies are classified below into three main areas: (1) selection and recruitment, (2) education and training, and (3) job performance.

Selection and Recruitment. Personnel shortages present a serious problem to the field of public health. As is true for the entire health area, there is an urgent need for additional trained personnel. According to a survey of 50 state official health agencies in 1956, "lack of adequate, well-trained personnel" was mentioned by more than half the sample as representing the most important problem.[36] This shortage of personnel is documented by the employment census of local health units conducted by the United States Public Health Service in 1960. According to the findings of this survey:

> ... In 1960, there were 610 (out of 1,557) local health units without a full-time physician, as compared to 522 units in 1958. An

additional 248 units employed less than 1 physician per 100,000 population.

... The extreme shortage of nurses is evidenced throughout local health jurisdictions. ... About 5 per cent had sufficient nurses on the staff to maintain a ratio of 1 nurse for every 5,000 population. Only 39 per cent of the units employed sufficient nurses to maintain a ratio of one nurse to 10,000 population.

... Less than one-fourth of the organizations had enough sanitation workers to provide at least 1 sanitarian for every 15,000 persons ... a desirable minimum goal.

... Less than 60 per cent of the reporting jurisdictions employed any professional or technical personnel other than physicians, nurses and sanitation workers.[37]

Not only do current shortages exist, but the situation appears to be growing worse rather than better. There are fewer physicians and engineers in public health today than there were in 1951, despite an increase in the population to be served. It is estimated by Anderson that there are fewer than half the physicians and nurses and not quite two-thirds of the sanitarians required to extend basic minimum health services throughout the United States.[38]

It is obvious from these statistics that studies of the recruitment of public health personnel offer a significant area for social research. Research is needed on who chooses or rejects public health work, why and how the decision is reached, what images and expectations of public health work exist, and what actual satisfactions and dissatisfactions are encountered on the job. These studies can provide valuable information on the various channels of entry into the public health field, the positive and negative features of public health work, the occupational attitudes and values of public health workers, and the development of one's self-identity and commitment to the field of public health.

Several studies dealing with the topics mentioned above have been conducted in the public health field, although these have been largely limited to the more professional groups of physicians and nurses. Back and his colleagues have studied medical students to determine their reasons for selecting or rejecting public health as a career.[39] Their findings show that public health is a deviant and secondary choice among the medical specialties. Other results indicate that students favorably disposed toward public health are more likely than students unfavorably disposed to come from low-income families and are less likely to count on their families for help in getting established in medical practice; their fathers are more likely to be in professions other than medicine and less likely to be in business; they are less likely to value independence of action, prestige within the profession, and a high income, and are more likely to think of an ideal job as one that contributes to knowledge.

The relatively low prestige of public health among medical students can be seen from their description of the type of student interested in public health. They characterized the medical student interested in public health as being less independent, less interested in money, less creative, and less ambitious than his fellow students.

Fowler, in a study of 50 public health physicians who had completed a training program in public health, found that the choice of public health as a specialty created serious professional role conflicts for the young physician. To some extent, public health practice with its total community or group emphasis conflicted with the traditional, clinical, one-to-one doctor-patient relationship. Thus entrance into public health tended to suggest a rejection of medical practice and one's allegiance to the medical profession as such.[40]

A study of 1,129 public health workers in four state and local health departments by Cohart and Hiscock supports the picture of public health as a secondary choice among health personnel.[41] Only 17 per cent of the professional and semiprofessional public health workers started their careers in public health, with the average public health worker entering public health after having spent seven years in other fields. Half the physicians had been in private practice before entering public health. Undoubtedly, the increased professionalization of the public health field and the growth of governmental aid to training in the ten years since this study was made have increased the number of public health workers whose primary allegiance has been to public health, but it is probably still true that public health largely represents a secondary choice of occupation.

The reasons given by the public health workers in the Cohart and Hiscock study for entering the field of public health emphasize the current rather haphazard recruitment policies, with "chance" being the most prominent factor. Other reasons given included personal contacts, attraction of the work, and favorable working conditions.

The relative advantages and disadvantages of public health service as opposed to private practice are indicated by a survey of physicians in Puerto Rico, both in and out of government service.[42] The advantages of working for the government were perceived as: (1) retirement pensions, (2) vacations, (3) service to the community, (4) interesting work, (5) opportunity to study, (6) remuneration during the early years, and (7) more home life. Opposed to these were the advantages of private practice, listed as follows: (1) financial remuneration in the long run, (2) independence, (3) conditions of work, (4) relations with patients, (5) public prestige, (6) social position, (7) medical prestige, (8) feeling of accomplishment, and (9) sense of security.

This listing points to one of the most serious problems in recruitment of physicians to a career in public health—that of the greater prestige and higher financial remuneration currently enjoyed by private practice in the United States. It is doubtful that public health can successfully attract the kind of medical student who is seeking fame and fortune; rather it must concentrate on those future doctors who place a higher value on public service, regular hours, favorable working conditions, and job security.

Like the medical student, the nursing student must make a choice between private duty and institutional employment. Unlike physicians, however, the overwhelming proportion of nurses are to be found employed by institutions—nearly two-thirds of the 460,000 professional nurses in the United States.[43] Most of these nurses work in hospitals and related institutions, with only a small number, about 14,500, holding full-time jobs in health departments.

Perhaps more research has been done on the nursing occupation than on any other in the health field.[44] Recruitment of young girls to nursing is a serious matter—there is a major shortage of nursing personnel despite the fact that one out of every 16 girls who graduate from high school enters the nursing field. This shortage affects all branches of nursing, including public health.

For the most part, nursing as a public health profession presents an attractive picture to the young girl. In terms of occupational rankings, nursing compares favorably with teaching and social work.[45] A majority of girls agree that nursing is a calling which provides an excellent opportunity to render an important service to humanity.[46] Most surveys stress the importance of the humanitarian motive for high school girls considering nursing as a career. The desire to be a nurse originates early in life, with two-thirds of the nurses placing their decision to enter nursing before the age of sixteen.[47] An important factor in the choice of nursing for many lower social class girls is the opportunity it presents for an education and social mobility.[48]

Recruitment into nursing is largely a matter of personal influence. Middlewood found that almost half of the students she interviewed reported that they were favorably influenced by relatives who were nurses or doctors.[49] A majority of the nursing students in Puerto Rico state that their fathers and mothers exerted a positive influence upon them in their choice of nursing. For this group, having a friend who was a nurse or nursing student was most frequently agreed upon as having been important in their selection of nursing as a career.[50]

As in the case of the physicians in Puerto Rico, nurses there are more likely to be attracted to public health service than to private duty because of such advantages as regular hours of work, job security, paid vacations, and a retirement pension, and to be discouraged from entering public health nursing because of its lower public and professional prestige.[51] We lack similar information for the continental United States, but it seems likely that corresponding prestige problems exist for public health nursing. The highest status in all nursing is coming to be attached to the administrative responsibilities in hospital care.

It has been claimed that "the present function of the graduate nurse is not to nurse the patient, but to see that he is nursed."[52] One result has been the rapid growth of nonprofessional nursing personnel. Given the current scarcity of graduate nurses, it is doubtful that this trend can, or should, be reversed. It is beginning to find its way into public health nursing where public health assistants are currently being recruited to help overcome the shortage of public health nurses. It is quite likely that the future will see the further development of such nonprofessional nursing roles in public health, despite the objections of professional nurses who fear a loss in prestige. The long and hard fight of nurses for professional status has characterized the growth of the nursing profession and it is likely that any lowering of professional standards will be strongly resisted both inside and outside public health.

Education and Training. The educational background of public health workers reflects the secondary nature of public health work at present for most public health occupational groups. Since public health workers are "borrowed" from many diverse occupations to perform a wide variety of tasks, it is to be expected that their primary formal education will not be in the field of public health and that on-the-job training and experience will be of greater importance than in most professional fields.

In fact, only 10 per cent of the 1,129 public health workers in the four states surveyed by Cohart had graduate degrees in public health. However, an additional 23 per cent had taken undergraduate courses in public health or had a certificate in public health nursing. The public health training of 41 per cent of the workers had been limited to informal training only, and 26 per cent had no public health training whatsoever. To a large extent, the deficiency in formal training is compensated for by widespread in-service training programs, with half the public health workers having taken short courses in institutes, 30 per cent having undergone field training with other agencies, and 20 per cent having participated in official in-service training programs.[53]

Thus it is apparent that specialized training in public health is currently the exception rather than the rule. The need for increased training is emphasized by a United States Public Health Service survey in 1957, which estimated that while some 17,000 professional positions in state and local health departments call for graduate or specialized public health preparation, more than half or almost 9,000 persons in these positions have not had such training. This study concludes:

> Modern forces are reshaping public health philosophy and practice. . . . Postgraduate training and residencies in public health practice have become as essential to this medical specialty as to the clinical specialties.[54]

In 1948 preventive medicine and public health achieved recognition as a specialty by the American Medical Association with the establishment of the American Board of Preventive Medicine and Public Health. Residency training in the public health specialty follows the general pattern of approved clinical residency for any postgraduate training of physicians. The Master of Public Health degree from an accredited school of public health is required by the American Board of Preventive Medicine and Public Health for certification for Grade I-A and I-B health officers. In 1959–1960, a total of 1,660 students were enrolled in graduate schools of public health in the United States, of whom 750 received degrees—overwhelmingly the M.P.H. About one out of four of these graduate students in public health were medical doctors.[55]

The curriculum of these graduate schools of public health has been the subject of a great deal of debate. This controversy is significant insofar as it again raises the question of public health as a medical or administrative specialty. Generally, the core curriculum for the M.P.H. degree requires the student to take at least one comprehensive course in each of the following subjects: public health administration, biostatistics, sanitary science, and epidemiology. Additional required courses include such subjects as tropical medicine, labor relations, microbiology, nutrition, public health nursing, and occupational health. A recent trend is toward increased specialization, with separate public health degrees in industrial health, dental public health, tropical medicine, and hospital administration.

Underlying the public health curriculum debate are the changing nature of public health practice and the degree of importance to be assigned to training in the social sciences. More and more, the public health officer, as we shall see in the next section, is called upon to exercise interpersonal rather than technical skills and to make administrative rather than medical decisions. Perkins presents the problem in these words:

> We have heard that we need more use of the social and political sciences. I would like to raise that question regarding the training of the directors of local health departments. I think we have a right to, and should, look at current qualifications for directors of local health units, because it seems to me that either the M.D. must need a lot more training in the social sciences and administration than he got in my day, or perhaps we should evolve a new training program for these top administrators. Perhaps it ought to begin with individuals who are community-minded and community-oriented at the outset, rather than individual patient-interested as practically all medical students are.[56]

This challenge to current graduate education in public health is reflected in the responses of Cohart's sample of 1,129 public health workers. In evaluating their training in public health, only 26 per cent stressed the importance of learning "specific technical procedures," a figure which was almost matched by such social science subject matter as "interpersonal relations" (23 per cent), "knowledge of community" (18 per cent), and "administration" (15 per cent).[57] Fowler's study of public health officers supports this concern on the part of trainees with the learning of functional skills in administration and public relations.[58]

Fowler's study is particularly interesting from a sociological point of view because of its emphasis upon the significance of the graduate degree in public health for the physician. She raises the question of the meaning of the M.P.H. and Dr. P.H. degrees as symbols for an M.D.'s accolade or sinecure—a question that could be similarly raised for many other graduate professional degrees. According to her survey of 50 public health physicians with advanced degrees, these degrees serve an important "union card" function for entry into the higher-status public health positions. Fowler concludes as follows:

> Summing up its most rewarding value—and in the broadest terms —it seems that the School of Public Health year offered the symbols of a "union card," of "prestige," but, in addition, the "in-group" ex-

perience and knowledge which made possible a sense of transition into a new dimension of professional aptitude. It represented a "rite de passage" from one medical specialty—or the limited orientations of medical school—to another.[59]

The "rite de passage" aspect of medical training has received a great deal of attention from sociologists, although no similar studies have been conducted among public health students. Two major "socialization" studies have been carried out among medical students at Cornell University Medical College[60] and the University of Kansas Medical School.[61] The objective of these sociological studies of the medical school was to investigate the social and psychological environment offered by the medical school, and the bearing of that environment on the acquisition of knowledge, skills, attitudes, and values by medical students; and to observe the transformation in attitudes, values, and future plans that took place in medical students as they moved through the different phases of their professional training.

Given the divided loyalties of the public health professional to medicine and public health, a significant area for future social research might well involve this "socialization" process. Such a study could provide valuable insights into those factors facilitating or impeding the professionalization of the public health occupations and the development of an allegiance with and a pride in public health work. Such self-identifications are the hallmark of any professional field.

Job Performance. In a rapidly changing field that is characterized by as many different professional and nonprofessional tasks as public health, it is natural to find the definition of occupational statuses and roles subject to a great deal of flexibility. The allocation of specific duties and the manner in which these are to be carried out will vary from one public health agency to another, depending upon such factors as size and type of community to be served and the availability of trained personnel. In very few cases are job descriptions sufficiently standardized to permit any meaningful analysis of the quality and quantity of occupational performance.

Only two significant studies have been made of the allocation of the public health workers' time to programs and to specific functional categories of activity. One of these was conducted in Maryland, the other in Mississippi. In Mississippi, the amount of time devoted to different programs shows the following rank order: maternal and child health (36.5 per cent), environmental sanitation (28.1 per cent), acute communicable diseases (11.2 per cent), tuberculosis (10.1 per cent), venereal disease (9.7 per cent), and chronic disease (3.4 per cent).[62] The Maryland study reported a similar rank ordering of program activities, with approximately one-third of the time being spent in performing technical or direct service activities, one-third in administration and community relations and organization, and the remaining one-third in ancillary services.[63] The Maryland study also reported that the medical personnel particularly tended to spend more time in administration and community activities and less time in direct services. The amount of time devoted to administration as a whole and its major subcategories increased as the level of education, amount of public health training, and salary increased.[64]

The Maryland study is interesting for its attempt to determine the satisfactions and dissatisfactions of public health workers with their jobs. In general, three out of five expressed satisfaction, while 14 per cent indicated that they were unhappy in their work. The most frequent sources of dissatisfaction concerned working conditions and salary, while the greatest satisfaction came from the contribution of public health to public welfare and from interpersonal relations with one's fellow workers.

These findings are supported by a number of studies of nursing personnel that substantiate the general picture of public health as a field in which the work is gratifyingly significant but the working conditions and salary are causes of discontent. In general, public health nursing enjoys higher prestige than hospital nursing, probably because of its more independent status. A study of public health nurses in Michigan reported that the major source of job satisfaction for the public health nurse related to the work she was doing with children, with families and with community groups, while the unsatisfactory aspect of her work stemmed from working conditions, especially time-consuming activities which she believed did not require public health nursing skills.[65]

Several studies have characterized the transition from student nurse to practicing nurse as one of "disillusionment" as the technical-administrative functions of routine nursing activity overshadowed the sense of any personal contribution to patient welfare.[66]

A great deal of research has been devoted to the determination of nursing functions and activities. Historically, it is instructive to note that the problem of the most effective organization of nursing services was the subject of a great deal of research in the 1920's and 1930's when public health nursing was in its infancy, while today the focus of research has shifted from specifying tasks to defining roles and statuses, perhaps marking the emergence of nursing as a professional activity.

Foremost among the early studies dealing with the organization of nursing services was the Commonwealth Fund study of public health nursing, administration, and practice.[67] The purpose of this study, conducted in 1931–1932, was to evaluate the state of public health nursing at the time and to compare variations in the organization of public health services. Information was collected from 28 different communities on the distribution and administrative control of nursing services, the types of services being rendered, the qualifications of personnel, working conditions, community relationships, and so forth. A comparison of nursing performance showed "bedside care" ranking high in quality, while "teaching" ranked low. One of the major recommendations made then, and one that is still being made, called for the greater integration of nursing services in the community through the use of combination agencies.

These early studies of public health nursing were greatly concerned with describing the functions of the public health nurse. Nursing staffs kept detailed records of the time distribution of their activities, including field visits, medical and nursing conferences, school service, community organization, and clerical tasks. The time analysis showed that between 50 and 60 per cent of the total working time of a public health nurse was devoted to professional tasks, while the remainder was spent on other duties.[68]

Following these early studies on nursing services and functions, there was an increasing concern with the professional role and status of nurses.[69] The later studies were devoted to exploring the "image" of nurses—their own and the public's perception and definition of nursing, and the professional standing of nurses. This research showed the importance of such images and definitions to the nurse as reflected in her choice of and satisfaction with the profession and also its importance as evaluated by the public. Inadequate definitions of appropriate and acceptable nursing functions and behavior underlie many of the current resistances to changes in public health nursing roles, especially the resistance to the introduction of nonprofessional public health nursing assistants.[70]

While no studies comparable to those of nurses have been made of public health physicians, there are several studies currently under way of the changing role of the public health officer. These studies are particularly interesting because of their emphasis upon the conflict between the medical and social aspects of public health work. With tradition and prestige on the side of the medical, the public health officer who finds the largest proportion of his time devoted to nonmedical tasks faces a professional dilemma. This dilemma includes not only a mixed allegiance to medical versus administrative science but an even more troublesome conflict between private and "social" medicine.

Cohart and Hiscock in their analysis of the amount of time public health officers devoted to various activities found that the largest proportion of time was spent on administrative work and community relations and organization.[71] Wellin and Levine, in an analysis of the health officer's role, find this role to be quite complicated and to contain a number of inherent sources of conflict. They discern the health officer as functioning in four different capacities: health administrator, public official, physician, and community leader. In fulfilling these roles, he must maintain working relationships with a wide variety of health personnel, including other public health physicians and public health workers, other members of the medical profession, and the personnel of various community organizations, voluntary agencies, and other public agencies. Each of these groups has somewhat different expectations of the health officer's skills and responsibilities, which often lead to conflicting demands.[72]

This disparity in the image of the public health officer is documented by the detailed case studies of Fowler in her research on public health physicians. The public health officer offers three different images to the public and to his colleagues: a "doctor" image of the medical specialist in professional practice, an "administrator" image of the public servant who runs a bureaucratic organization, and a "community leader" image of the organizer and educator who provides guidance and assistance in community health activities. He thus becomes doctor-administrator-community leader who must function as a kind of "community medicine man."[73]

A current study by the Harvard University School of Public Health on the interrelationships of the various health agencies in a New England community stresses the role of the health officer as a key agent in the exchange of three main elements of community health: clients, labor services, and resources other than labor.[74] This study has revealed that a crucial problem facing health officers is the development of effective working relationships with other official and voluntary organizations. Modern public health practice is strongly dependent upon community support and cooperation, as we have seen in the previous chapter.

We know very little at present about the image which various segments of the public hold about public health functions, organizations, or personnel. Probably, as Roney maintains, "Public health people have been confused with policemen, S.P.C.A. officials, social welfare personnel, street sweepers, garbage collectors, private duty nurses, practicing physicians and others."[75] In view of the importance of public cooperation in public health activities, we need to know much more about the myths, prejudices, stereotypes, fantasies, and projections which the various health services and personnel arouse, and the functions these serve for the public.

The ambiguity in regard to public health occupational roles extends even to health personnel themselves. A study of the perceptions of public health physicians, nurses, and educators of each other showed disagreement not only among the different occupational groups but also within each group concerning their major functions. Differences in role perception appear to be greatest for public health nurses and least for health educators. Ambiguity was most pronounced in regard to which of the three groups was most likely to carry out activities requiring predominantly interpersonal skills and occurred more frequently in regard to internal, integrative activities than to activities directed toward external goals.[76] To a large extent, these relatively unclear definitions of public health roles are probably a reflection of the current developmental stage of public health work.

At the present time, we also lack studies of professional-client relationships for public health workers and the people they serve, such as exist for medical practitioners and their patients. This area offers some interesting possibilities for research on barriers to effective utilization of public health services by the public. The physician-patient relationship in the public health clinic, the public health nurse-family relationship in the home, the sanitarian-restauranteur or landlord relationship, the health educator-community group relationship, and so on present highly significant problems of role definition, communication, and interaction for public health work. The increasing part played by official health agencies in the area of medical care makes such studies of interpersonal relations in the public health field particularly timely.

The need for social research on both the organizational and occupational problems in public health discussed above is underscored by the responses of a sample of 50 health officials who were asked by the National Health Council, "What are the most important problems you are now facing (or anticipating) in the extension or modification of community health services?" At the top of the list were problems in organizational financing (56 per cent), lack of adequate, well-trained personnel (52 per cent), and lack of coordination of public health activities in the community (40 per cent).[77] The rapid growth and expanding programs of public health have created new problems of organization and personnel which require a radical reformulation of public health services. As evaluated by Perkins:

> This whole matter of establishing and revamping local health departments is becoming increasingly complex. Gone are the days of

the neat package of the county health department—For Sale: at X dollars, 50,000 population, one M.D. health officer with one year post-graduate training in a school of public health, one sanitary engineer, one supervising nurse and ten public health nurses, or some such package.[78]

It is difficult to foresee what the organizational and occupational structure of the field of public health will be in the future. The many new developments discussed in Chapter II will make their mark upon the traditional organization and staffing of public health units. Public health today is in an era of ferment, experimentation, and change, and most certainly to be affected will be current administrative arrangements and occupational groupings.

NOTES TO CHAPTER VI

1. Straus, Robert, "The Nature and Status of Medical Sociology," *American Sociological Review*, vol. 22, April, 1957, p. 203.
2. Sanders, Irwin T., "Public Health in the Community" in Freeman, Howard, Sol Levine, and Leo G. Reeder, *Handbook of Medical Sociology*. Prentice-Hall, Inc., Englewood Cliffs, N. J., 1963, pp. 369–396.
3. Foster, George, "Public Health and Behavioral Science: The Problems of Teamwork," *American Journal of Public Health*, vol. 51, September, 1961, p. 1292.
4. Mountin, Joseph W., Evelyn Flook, and Edward E. Minty, *Distribution of Health Services in the Structure of State Government, 1950*. U.S. Public Health Service, Publication No. 184, Part I, Government Printing Office, Washington, 1952.
5. Wellin, Edward, and Milvoy S. Seacat, "Social Science in the Health Field: A Review of Research (1954-1959)," *American Journal of Public Health*, vol. 52, September, 1962, pp. 1465–1472.
6. *Hospitals*, vol. 35, August, 1961. Guide Issue.
7. Burling, Temple, Edith Lentz, and Robert N. Wilson, *The Give and Take in Hospitals*. G. P. Putnam's Sons, New York, 1956.
8. Smith, Harvey L., "Two Lines of Authority: The Hospital's Dilemma," *The Modern Hospital*, vol. 84, March, 1955, pp. 59–64.
9. Coser, Rose L., "Authority and Decision-Making in a Hospital," *American Sociological Review*, vol. 23, February, 1958, pp. 56–63.
10. Stanton, Alfred H., and Morris S. Schwartz, *The Mental Hospital:* A Study of Institutional Participation in Psychiatric Illness and Treatment. Basic Books, Inc., New York, 1954.
11. Rosen, George, and Edward Wellin, "A Bookshelf on the Social Sciences and Public Health," *American Journal of Public Health*, vol. 49, April, 1959, pp. 441–454.
12. Greve, Clifford H., and Josephine R. Campbell, *Organization and Staffing for Local Health Services*. Rev. ed., U.S. Public Health Service, Publication No. 682, Government Printing Office, Washington, 1961.

13. Atwater, Reginald M., "A New Generation—A New Ferment," Foreword to "A Critique of Community Health Services," *American Journal of Public Health*, vol. 47, part 2, November, 1957, p. v.
14. Mountin, Joseph W., and Evelyn Flook, *Guide to Health Organization in the United States, 1951.* U.S. Public Health Service, Publication No. 196, Government Printing Office, Washington, 1953, p. 60.
15. Roemer, Milton I., and E. A. Wilson, *Organized Health Services in a County of the United States.* U.S. Public Health Service, Publication No. 197, Government Printing Office, Washington, 1952.
16. Connery, Robert H., and others, *Mental Health in Metropolitan Areas:* A Pilot Study. A Report to the Surgeon General's Committee on Mental Health Activities. Mimeographed, n.d.
17. Donabedian, Avedis, and S. J. Axelrod, "Organizing Medical Care Programs to Meet Health Needs," *Annals of the American Academy of Political and Social Science*, vol. 337, September, 1961, p. 55. This entire issue is devoted to the topic "Meeting Health Needs by Social Action."
18. Etzioni, Amitai, "New Directions in the Study of Organizations and Society," *Social Research*, vol. 27, Summer, 1960, pp. 223–228.
19. Johns, Ray E., and David F. de Marche, *Community Organization and Agency Responsibility.* Association Press, New York, 1951.
20. Levine, Sol, and Paul White, "Exchange as a Conceptual Framework for the Study of Interorganizational Relationships," *Administrative Science Quarterly*, vol. 5, March, 1961, pp. 583–601.
21. Hamlin, Robert H., "The Role of Voluntary Agencies in Meeting the Health Needs of Americans," *Annals of the American Academy of Political and Social Science*, vol. 337, September, 1961, pp. 93–102.
22. Levine, Sol, and Paul White, "The Community of Health Organizations" in Freeman, Levine, and Reeder, editors, *op. cit.*, pp. 321–347.
23. Dixon, James P., "Development Problems of Official Services in Keeping in Time with the Times," *American Journal of Public Health*, vol. 47, part 2, November, 1957, p. 18.
24. National Advisory Health Council, *Medical Care in the United States.* U.S. Public Health Service, Government Printing Office, Washington, March, 1961, p. 32.
25. Demerath, Nicholas J., "The Place of the Sciences of Administration in Medical Care." Paper presented at the Annual Meeting of the American Association for the Advancement of Science, Denver, Colorado, December, 29, 1961.
26. Cornely, Paul B., and Stanley K. Bigman, *Cultural Considerations in Changing Health Attitudes.* Howard University, Washington, December, 1961, p. 170. Mimeographed.
27. Simmel, Arnold, and David B. Ast, "Some Correlates of Opinion on Fluoridation," *American Journal of Public Health*, vol. 52, August, 1962, pp. 1272–1273.
28. Ennes, Howard, "Toward a Constructive Appraisal of Community Health Services," *American Journal of Public Health*, vol. 47, part 2, November, 1957, p. 5.
29. Rosenau, Milton Joseph, "Courses and Degrees in Public Health Work," *Journal of the American Medical Association*, vol. 64, March 6, 1915, p. 794.
30. Greve, Clifford H., and Josephine R. Campbell, *op. cit.*, p. 44.
31. Baumgartner, Leona, "Relationships of Public Health and Organized Medicine." Address to Florida Public Health Association, September 24, 1959.
32. Committee on Professional Education, "Public Health Degrees and Certificates Granted in the United States and Canada During the Academic Year 1939–40," *American Journal of Public Health*, vol. 30, December, 1940, p. 1456.

33. Troupin, James L., "Schools of Public Health in the United States and Canada: 1959–1960," *American Journal of Public Health*, vol. 50, November, 1960.
34. Parran, Thomas, "Committee on Professional Education," *American Journal of Public Health*, vol. 51, March, 1961, pp. 471–473.
35. Croog, Sydney, "Interpersonal Relations in Medical Settings" in Freeman, Levine, and Reeder, editors, *op. cit.*, pp. 241–271. This chapter contains an excellent analysis of occupational roles in medical settings.
36. "A Critique of Community Public Health Services," *American Journal of Public Health*, vol. 47, part 2, November, 1957, p. 40.
37. Greve, Clifford H., and Josephine R. Campbell, *op. cit.*, pp. 38–43.
38. Anderson, Otis L., "Training Opportunities for Public Health Personnel," *Public Health Reports*, vol. 72, August, 1957, p. 681.
39. Back, Kurt W., and others, "Public Health as a Career of Medicine: Secondary Choice Within a Profession," *American Sociological Review*, vol. 23, October, 1958, pp. 533–541. See also Coker, R. E., and others, "Public Health as Viewed by the Medical Student," *American Journal of Public Health*, vol. 49, May, 1959, pp. 601–609.
40. Fowler, Manet, *Evaluation of Public Health Physician Training*. New York State Department of Health, Progress Report, February, 1959. Mimeographed.
41. Cohart, Edward M., and Ira V. Hiscock, "A Profile of the Public Health Worker," *American Journal of Public Health*, vol. 45, December, 1955, pp. 1525–1532. See also Cohart, E., W. Willard, and I. Hiscock, "The Yale Study in Public Health Administration," *Public Health Reports*, vol. 70, May, 1955, p. 452.
42. *Medical and Hospital Care in Puerto Rico:* A Report Submitted to the Governor and the Legislature of the Commonwealth of Puerto Rico by the School of Public Health and Administrative Medicine. Columbia University, and the Department of Health of Puerto Rico, February, 1962, pp. 141–148.
43. *Facts About Nursing*. American Nurses' Association, New York, 1960.
44. Corwin, Ronald G., and Marvin J. Taves, "Nursing and Other Health Professions" in Freeman, Levine, and Reeder, editors, *op. cit.*, pp. 187–212.
45. Bullock, Robert P., *What Do Nurses Think of Their Profession?* The Ohio State University Research Foundation, Columbus, Ohio, 1954, pp. 27–62.
46. Taves, Marvin J., and Ronald G. Corwin, *The Image of Nursing Among High School Girls*. Ohio State University, Bureau of Business Research. In preparation.
47. Williams, Robin M., and Rose K. Goldsen, *Selection or Rejection of Nursing as a Career*. Cornell University, Ithaca, N. Y., 1960.
48. Hughes, Everett C., Helen M. Hughes, and Irwin Deutscher, *Twenty Thousand Nurses Tell Their Story*. J. B. Lippincott Co., Philadelphia, 1958.
49. Middlewood, Esther L., "Why Do Students Drop Out?" *American Journal of Nursing*, vol. 46, December, 1946, pp. 838–840.
50. *Medical and Hospital Care in Puerto Rico*, p. 157. (See note 42.)
51. *Ibid.*, pp. 164–165.
52. Saunders, Lyle, "The Changing Role of Nurses," *American Journal of Nursing*, vol. 54, September, 1954, pp. 1094–1098.
53. Cohart, Edward M., and Ira V. Hiscock, *op. cit.*, p. 1527.
54. Anderson, Otis L., *op. cit.*, p. 682.
55. Troupin, James L., *op. cit.*, pp. 18–19.
56. Perkins, James E., "Community Organization," *American Journal of Public Health*, vol. 47, November, 1957, part 2, p. 24.

57. Cohart, Edward M., and Ira V. Hiscock, *op. cit.*, p. 1526.
58. Fowler, Manet, *op. cit.*, p. 7.
59. Fowler, Manet, *M.P.H., Dr. P. H. Degrees—Symbols for an M.D.'s Accolade or Sinecure?* New York State Department of Health. Mimeographed, n.d.
60. Merton, Robert K., George G. Reader, and Patricia L. Kendall, editors, *The Student Physician.* Harvard University Press, Cambridge, 1957.
61. Becker, Howard, and others, *Boys in White:* Student Culture in Medical School. University of Chicago Press, Chicago, 1961.
62. Milne, J. A., and others, "Time Study of Public Health Activities in Mississippi," *Public Health Reports*, vol. 68, April, 1953, pp. 378–390.
63. Cohart, Edward M., and Ira V. Hiscock, *op. cit.*, p. 1530.
64. Cohart, Edward M., and W. R. Willard, "Functional Distribution of Working Time in Five County Health Departments," *Public Health Reports*, vol. 70, July, 1955, p. 716.
65. Kellogg, Winifred, "What Public Health Nurses Like About Their Jobs," *Public Health Reports*, vol. 72, February, 1957, pp. 121–125.
66. Corwin, Ronald G., Marvin J. Taves, and J. Eugene Haas, "Professional Disillusionment," *Nursing Research*, vol. 10, Summer, 1961, pp. 141–144.
67. Tucker, Katherine, and Hortense Hilbert, *Survey of Public Health Nursing, Administration and Practice.* The Commonwealth Fund, New York, 1934.
68. Winslow, Emma A., "The Measurement of Nurse-Power," *Public Health Nurse*, vol. 19, October, 1927, pp. 492–498. See also Winslow, Emma, "More About the Measurement of Nurse Power," *Public Health Nurse*, vol. 20, February, 1928.
69. Saunders, Lyle, *op. cit.* (See note 52.)
70. Reissman, Leonard, and John H. Rohrer, editors, *Change and Dilemma in the Nursing Profession.* G. P. Putnam's Sons, New York, 1957.
71. Cohart, Edward M., and Ira V. Hiscock, *op. cit.*, p. 1529.
72. Wellin, Edward, and Sol Levine, "The Role of the Health Officer: A Sociological Inquiry." Paper presented to the Committee on Preventive Medicine and Social Science, Social Science Research Council, 1960.
73. Fowler, Manet, "Image and Experience," New York State Department of Health, 1960. Dittoed.
74. Levine, Sol, and Paul White, *op. cit.* (See note 20.)
75. Roney, James G., *Public Health for Reluctant Communities.* James G. Roney, New York, 1961, pp. 22–23. Privately printed.
76. Arnold, Mary F., "Perception of Professional Role Activities in the Local Health Department," *Public Health Reports*, vol. 77, January, 1962, pp. 80–88.
77. Ennes, Howard, editor, "A Critique of Community Public Health Services," *American Journal of Public Health*, vol. 47, November, 1957, part 2, p. 40.
78. Perkins, James E., *op. cit.*, p. 22.

VII

ACTIVITIES OF SOCIOLOGISTS IN PUBLIC HEALTH

IN PREVIOUS CHAPTERS we have dealt with the relationship of sociology as a discipline to public health. We now shift our focus to the professional representatives of this discipline—the sociologists—and discuss some of the characteristics, activities, and problems of sociologists entering the field of public health today. Our main emphasis will be upon the unique contribution that sociologists "qua" sociologists can and do make to public health. Sociologists in public health may find themselves performing a great many valuable functions that are only remotely related to their training or skills as a sociologist. But for us the major question will be, "What can sociologists do that others can't do?" although we will examine the question, "What do sociologists do that nonsociologists can do as well but don't, or won't?"

Several analyses have been made of the role of social scientists in the health field. Most of these pertain only to social scientists working in medical settings, for example, the paper by Bloom and associates on sociologists in medical schools,[1] and have limited value for our present problem. A comprehensive review has been made by Wellin for the National Institute of Mental Health and probably represents the most intensive investigation to date.[2] A valuable contribution to our understanding of the relationship of behavioral scientists to public health is the *Report of the Surgeon General's Ad Hoc Committee on Mental Health Activities*. The United States Public Health Service, in concerning itself with the relations between mental health and the rest of public health, is also becoming seriously interested in the broad role of the behavioral sciences in public health.[3] In general, however, much of our knowledge about the problems of sociologists working in public health is based upon personal accounts of individual sociologists and there is a great need for more systematic research in this area.

By and large, sociologists may be found in three main areas of public health—research, teaching, and service. At present, research is probably the most frequent form of endeavor, with teaching in second place but rapidly increasing in importance, while service or operational activities constitute only a negligible proportion of the sociological effort. This distribution reflects the current state of need, with the greatest demand being for sociologists to study the many unanswered questions about community and individual behavior facing public health today. By tradition, public health has turned to research when faced with new problems, and, given this orientation, it is not surprising that public health has looked to the sociologist primarily for his skills in doing research on social health problems. To a lesser extent, and perhaps more a token recognition of the need than a determined effort to meet it, public health has also asked the sociologist to teach and train its own professional students in social science knowledge and methods. Undoubtedly, this differential emphasis also reflects the ease with which a health research project can be initiated and integrated into ongoing activities, as opposed to the rather more difficult task of introducing a new teaching program into an established and crowded professional curriculum.

Finally, in regard to service activities, very few sociologists today are actively engaged in the operational aspects of public health programs. On the one hand, this type of function calls for an intimate knowledge of public health practice—knowledge that can be obtained only by professional training in public health and by actual work on the job. On the other hand, sociologists are not likely by selection, training, and temperament to be interested in service programs. They tend to be "thinkers" and not "doers." However, as social research on public health problems contributes proven knowledge, and as both social science and public health students receive training in both social science and public health, we may expect to see a new breed of public health practitioner whose specific job it will be to apply social science knowledge to the operation of routine public health programs. Hawkins suggests that a major need in the application of social science to operating health programs today is for "generalists" who "aspire to generality and are willing to undertake the discomforts, anxieties and occasional disappointments required to achieve generality."[4]

The 1961 survey of medical sociologists by the Health Information Foundation provides substantiating data on the relative frequency of research, teaching, and service activities among sociologists in the health field. While the survey was not limited to public health, these differences are large enough to justify their probable accuracy for public health alone. Overwhelmingly, research was the main activity of this group, with 82 per cent of the sample engaged in it. Somewhat fewer than half were teaching at least part-time, while only one-fourth were involved in any administrative functions. Asked which activities they *preferred*, the majority mentioned research first and teaching second, with consultation and administration being mentioned only rarely as primary interests.[5] When one considers the overwhelming service orientation of the field of public health, it is obvious that sociologists entering public health today do not see themselves as public health workers but rather as researchers and teachers.

Partly because of this discrepancy between the needs of public health and the desires of sociologists, and partly because of the absence of any clear-cut career lines and the inevitable conflicts of cross-disciplinary work (which is more likely to be the case), public health is a highly marginal area for most sociologists. One consequence that deserves careful consideration in evaluating current accomplishments of sociology applied to public health is the probably poorer quality of sociologists now represented in public health. As was pointed out in a survey of sociologists in public health:

> This (high demand and low supply), plus the fact that the health field is still nearer the margin than the center of employment acceptable to qualified people, increases the risk that marginal or poorly-trained social scientists will be recruited.[6]

A sociologist leaving the tried and true paths of the academic world must face many frustrating, even if ultimately rewarding, experiences in a public health world of differing values and behaviors, as we shall see in the following chapter. Combined with these difficulties of daily existence is an often insecure financial underpinning, which gives some truth to the saying, "Soft money attracts only soft sociologists." In addition, there is often an isolation and lack of interaction with one's professional colleagues, which may engender a feeling of being "forgotten." There are certain safeguards which we will discuss next, but here we would like only to indicate some of the understandable drawbacks for a sociologist entering the public health field and to make the point that, in all probability, the best talents of sociology are not being applied to public health. In any evaluation of current accomplishments of sociology in public health this fact merits consideration.

Research Activities

We have already noted in the previous chapters the many areas of research on public health problems open to the sociologist. In general, the field of public health is highly research oriented. This applies not only to the university but also to the operating health agency, especially on the state and federal levels.

An increasingly large proportion of public health research takes place outside the laboratory or clinic in the field or community. As pictured by James, "What the laboratory bench is to the virologist, what the medical ward is to the clinical researcher, every single community can be to an inquiring health officer."[7]

As soon as public health research moved out of the laboratory, it entered upon the natural research ground of the social sciences. Sociological methods and techniques have been developed for, and are uniquely applicable to, the study of individuals, groups, and communities. As we have seen, social surveys, including the "panel technique" for longitudinal study, constitute a basic approach for public health to the study of the etiology and epidemiology of disease, the health status and responses of the individual, and the information, attitudes, and behavior of the public regarding public health programs. Community study techniques are directly applicable to the analysis of community forces affecting the support and utilization of health services. The comparative method of social research offers the necessary conceptual and technical knowledge for the conduct of cross-national health studies. The methodology of the sociological field experiment relates directly to the need of public health to evaluate the effectiveness of its services by means of demonstration programs and field trials. Demography and ecology, as well as social statistics, have a longer history in social science than in public health.

The established techniques of social research are rapidly becoming the accepted tools of modern public health research. The field of sociology has devoted many years of methodological research to such data-gathering problems as questionnaire construction, interviewing, sampling, and community observation, and to such equally important problems in the interpretation of data as the analysis of multiple variables, scale analysis and index construction, qualitative analysis, and content analysis. Problems in the design of research dealing with human populations, the determination of the reliability and validity of their responses, the measurement and prediction of their behavior are only some of the methodological areas of sociological sophistication that are occupying more and more of the time and attention of the public health research worker. It is easy to understand why public health has turned to sociologists for research personnel, and why sociologists have been attracted to research on public health problems. It is difficult to imagine a more natural alliance.

Analysis of the research activities of a number of health departments reveals a wide range of social science programs. Boek classifies these into five types as follows: (1) the evaluation of various current programs to determine whether or not expected goals are being reached; (2) appraisal of proposed programs; (3) the determination of relative values of different public health programs; (4) the discovering and/or developing of new, improved methods for meeting health problems and human needs; (5) a critical analysis in relation to function of the formal and informal structure of health department organization, including channels and media of communication and decision-making machinery.[8]

Social research activities are currently being carried on in almost all types of health agencies. On the federal level, social research in a public health context is to be found mainly in the Public Health Service, especially the National Institute of Mental Health, although sociologists are also represented in the Children's Bureau and the Office of Vocational Rehabilitation. Almost all state health departments secure part-time consultation from social researchers, with California, Colorado, Connecticut, Florida, Kentucky, Maryland, New Mexico, New York, Pennsylvania, and Washington employing full-time social scientists. Recently several city and county health departments have added full-time social scientists to their staffs, notably New York, Philadelphia, Los Angeles, Cambridge, and St. Louis County. All of these positions have been created within the past ten years.[9]

Social research on public health problems is an important part of the research programs of most of the schools of public health and constitutes an appreciable segment of research in medical schools and other universities. Under the research grants program of the National Institutes of Health, social research on public health problems has been receiving increasingly strong support. A major grant of several million dollars has recently been made to The University of Michigan School of Public Health for the development of evaluation studies under a program headed jointly by a public health professional and a behavioral scientist.

The 1957 survey by the Health Information Foundation offers some informative statistics concerning behavioral scientists doing research in the health field.[10] Research activities have taken two directions—research on the distribution of disease according to population characteristics, and research on the sociopsychological aspects of the provision and receipt of care. The newness of social research in the field of public health is indicated by the fact that almost 60 per cent of the respondents had received their degrees within the past six years (82 per cent were Ph.D.'s) and that 53 per cent had been in the health field two years or less.

The following table, reproduced from the Health Information Foundation report, is interesting as an indication of where this research was being done.

Agency	Per cent
University or college	67
Federal government	7
Research agencies (bureaus of social research in universities)	7
State and local governments	7
Foundations	4
Hospitals, clinics, and the like	3
Voluntary health and welfare agencies	2
Other	3
Total	100

This study reported that almost half of the behavioral scientists within universities and colleges were based in departments of sociology and anthropology. They also found some dual appointments although these were extremely rare. Foundations were given as a chief source of financial support, followed by the federal government.

In general, the social scientists doing research in the field of health expressed favorable attitudes toward their work, with 77 per cent anticipating as much or more research activity in the health field in the future as at present. Only 6 per cent felt their status had been affected unfavorably, while 68 per cent thought their status had been favorably affected. The following advantages were mentioned most often as being offered by research in the health field:

> The opportunity to apply, test, and develop behavioral science knowledge, theory, methodology, and hypotheses (62 per cent).
>
> The opportunity to deal with problems of vital importance to human welfare (39 per cent).
>
> Desirable working conditions and professional opportunities, such as employment security, financial reward, and so on (24 per cent).

The disadvantages of working in the health field were classified as follows:

> Lack of recognition of behavioral science as a legitimate scientific discipline in the health field and differences in status between behavioral scientists and medical personnel (36 per cent).

Isolation of the behavioral scientist from his parent discipline and danger of becoming a "quasi" expert (29 per cent).

Ignorance or misconception of the behavioral scientist's role in and contribution to the health field (19 per cent).

Lack of medical knowledge or understanding of the organization and structure of the health field by behavioral scientists (13 per cent).

There is every reason to believe that the trend in the six years since this survey was made has continued to be favorable toward research by social scientists in the health field. A more recent survey of medical sociologists in 1961 revealed that over two-thirds of the respondents believed that work in the health field had affected their professional careers favorably. About three-fourths said they liked working in the health field "a great deal."

This survey also asked the respondents about work settings. The five work settings most frequently mentioned were research units attached to universities, state or local government agencies, hospitals, medical schools, and graduate schools. Preferences of work settings were expressed, first, for research units attached to universities, second, for graduate schools, and, third, for medical schools. In all cases, however, only from about one-third to one-half were actually working in the setting they preferred.[11]

In an analysis of 565 social science research projects in the health field from 1954 to 1959, Wellin and Seacat found the following distribution of research according to the general subject matter being studied.

I. *Social Factors in Disease and Health (291)*
   a) Social factors in etiology, and distribution (125)
   b) Response and adjustment to disease (50)
   c) Attitudes related to disease (45)
   d) The therapeutic process (43)
   e) Health levels and health needs (16)
   f) Relation of disease to various social problems (12)

II. *Social factors in the Organization of Medical Care (274)*
   a) Services and facilities (93)
   b) Personnel (91)
   c) Social systems (90)

These 565 research projects were being conducted by a wide variety of agencies, which could be classified into five broad types: professional schools; social science and other academic departments; federal, state, and local government agencies; voluntary or service-type agencies; and research agencies. The authors note the surprisingly large role in health research of the traditionally service oriented agencies, both in terms of financing such research and in actually conducting research projects themselves.[12]

The rapid expansion of social research in the field of public health has resulted in a work situation characterized by exciting new opportunities for significant research, many large-scale projects of a scope only rarely before afforded the social sciences, collaborative work with non-social scientists, uncertain organizational affiliations and career lines, and a major emphasis upon tentative commitments. Undoubtedly, the currently high degree of opportunism and instability will give way to more systematic, planned, and secure working arrangements as the status and role relationships of social scientists in public health become more firmly established. For the present, however, as we shall see in the next chapter, there are many serious problems of communication and interaction.

Teaching Activities

The teaching of sociological concepts and methods relevant to public health and preventive medicine has benefited greatly from the general growth of interest on the part of medical schools in a more comprehensive approach to medical care. From this point of view, prevention and treatment are regarded as part of the same total health process, and the patient is seen not as a single individual, but as someone who is closely related to his family, friends, and community. This comprehensive, community-minded approach to health problems and medical care forms the basis for much of the current demand for sociological teaching in medicine and public health.

In an excellent analysis of current efforts at introducing social science teaching into medical and public health schools, a panel of sociologists and a medical educator points out:

Much of the history of medical school curricula during the past thirty years can be written in terms of an expanded effort to deal with the social aspects of medicine, usually within departments of psychiatry or preventive medicine. . . . Increased understanding of the etiology of disease—and the development of effective techniques of intervention—made prevention a possibility as well as a goal in medicine. The public health worker soon discovered that the successful introduction of preventive measures involved changing the customs and attitudes of whole communities.[13]

The trend toward the introduction of sociological content into public health and medical education is a reflection of the changing nature of health problems as discussed in Chapter III. The growth in importance of the chronic diseases and behavioral disorders with their intimate relationship to social factors in etiology and treatment, the increased complexity of medical care practices and administration, the shift from legislative control to voluntary participation in preventive programs, and the greater responsibility of community leadership and organization for the support of health programs have magnified the relevance of social forces in the control of disease and the conduct of public health programs. To prepare the public health profession to meet these changing problems of public health practice, sociologists, anthropologists, and psychologists have been recruited for teaching and on-the-job training of public health workers.

The rapidity of the growth of interest of public health in sociological training can be seen from a recent report on schools of public health in the United States. As of 1959–1960, there were 29 social scientists on the faculties of the 12 graduate schools of public health—12 full-time, 10 part-time, and 7 full-time in the university and part-time in the school of public health.[14] This expansion has been paralleled among medical and nursing schools, with about half of the 85 medical schools and an increasing number of the schools of nursing seeking the direct participation of social scientists in their teaching program.[15] A study of 70 medical schools in the United States revealed a total of 96 sociologists with faculty appointments, 33 being full-time, as compared to 583 psychologists, 408 of whom had full-time appointments, and 69 anthropologists of whom 29 were on a full-time basis. Thus, even though the number of sociologists in medical colleges has increased rapidly in the past ten years, it does not approach the number of psychologists similarly employed. Almost all of the sociologists are engaged in research, with fewer than half (46 per cent) giving formal classroom instruction.[16] The Health Information Foundation survey of medical sociologists reported that 44 per cent of the respondents were engaged in teaching activities, with an additional 33 per cent expressing the desire to do more teaching.[17]

Despite these encouraging figures of a widespread increase in importance of sociological instruction in schools of public health and medicine, it is important to recognize that social science courses are still very much on the periphery of public health and medical curricula. Their need may be recognized, but their place is not yet established. Public health, preventive medicine, and psychiatry, the departments within which the social sciences are most likely to be located, are themselves relatively low-status departments, and, to some extent, social science shares its problems of status and prestige with them. The majority of sociologists (60 per cent) in medical schools have appointments solely in departments of psychiatry.[18] Paul explains this affiliation in terms of the tightly constrained curricula of the medical schools, which have been slow to accept the behavioral sciences as part of the "basic" or preclinical sciences.[19] Jaco warns against this limited affiliation as harmful to the future development of sociology in medical education.[20]

One notable exception is the College of Medicine at the University of Kentucky, which has established a separate Department of Behavioral Science. This development has great significance for public health as well as medical education. As described by Straus:

> . . . The Department of Behavioral Science should be in a strong position to fulfill these major objectives: First, the delineation and synthesis of principles and content from the behavioral sciences which are specially pertinent to the understanding of human behavior in health and disease, and the correlation of these principles with those of the biological and physical sciences in the development of a conceptual frame of reference useful for the practice of comprehensive

medicine; Second, the application of behavioral science concepts and research findings to a further understanding of the diagnosis, treatment, and management of the individual patient, to the mobilization of health resources to meet the needs of society, and to the understanding of interpersonal relationships and social structure within medical institutions themselves.[21]

The objectives of this Department of Behavioral Science highlight the general content of most social science courses in medical and public health schools. In medical schools the accent is likely to be on the physician-patient relationship, while in schools of public health the major emphasis will be on the social and psychological factors affecting the success or failure of public health programs.

Paul makes a good case for the even greater relevance of social science content for the curricula of schools of public health than for medical schools. According to Paul, who has spent the past ten years building a program of social science teaching and research at the Harvard School of Public Health, public health schools differ from medical schools in five important respects—which affect positively the reception of social science teaching at schools of public health. First, schools of public health accent the promotion of good health and the prevention of disease rather than its treatment, thus calling for instruction on the nature of motivation, communication, and persuasion. Second, public health places greater emphasis on the community than on the individual, requiring a knowledge on the part of the public health student of such social science topics as group process, social organization, and cultural pattern. Third, the multi-disciplinary character of public health brings together students with a wide variety of disciplinary and professional backgrounds, offering the social science teacher a heterogeneous group usually with limited training in the social sciences. Fourth, public health students are largely postgraduate students and bring with them an awareness of the need to deal with problems in individual and community relations based upon actual experience. Fifth, schools of public health have a highly international student body with an understanding of the importance of cultural variations and a receptivity to a social science framework dealing with social and cultural factors.[22]

Despite this apparently natural convergence of social science and public health and the development of social science courses at almost all schools of public health, Troupin's survey revealed only two out of 750 graduates from schools of public health whose major subject was one of the behavioral sciences.[23] By and large, the social science teaching function is limited to the elementary, orientation type of course, although several schools of public health, notably Harvard, are beginning to offer integrated sequences of courses. Columbia is planning a program to train graduate social scientists for advanced degrees in social science and public health.

Examination of the catalogues of the various schools of public health reveals several types of course orientations: surveys of concepts of the social sciences relatively basic in orientation; somewhat proselytizing or propagandistic attempts to win enthusiasm for the social sciences among public health students; surveys of selected applications of social science theory or research methods to public health problems; and, finally, courses on the methods and techniques of social science research or more general scientific methodology.

For the most part, the teaching of social science in public health and medical schools consists of a combined sociology, social psychology, and social anthropology approach. Data, concepts, and theory are examined for their relevance to medicine and public health, rather than as social theory, per se. In this sense, the teaching is "applied" rather than "basic." One danger of this approach is that students do not receive a sufficient foundation in social science principles; they get only a brief "indoctrination" toward the relevance of social science to their professional field. The applied emphasis is probably inevitable in a professional school, but as Macgregor points out in relation to social science teaching in schools of nursing, this application must be preceded by the careful selection of a body of fundamental knowledge and then skillfully interwoven into the applied courses with an emphasis on synthesis and integration rather than dilution. She offers an interesting procedure for making social science teaching more effective by disseminating social science concepts into other aspects of the professional education. The social science content needs to be reinforced through use in other non-social science courses, largely through making the rest of the faculty aware of the social science aspects of their subject matter and encouraging them to apply this knowledge in their own teaching and supervision of students.[24] This integration, of course, is much to be desired, but extremely difficult to attain.

A good example of the possible integration of basic sociological concepts into the overall curriculum of the professional medical education, also applicable to public health, is offered by Straus in a discussion of what sociologists should teach in medical education.

> Emphasis on a number of concepts and approaches appears desirable in order to achieve these goals. First, the concept of health and medicine as a behavioral system should prove useful. Sociologists might stress the interrelationships of the following five behavior systems or systems of human adaptation: (a) internal body system, (b) the environmental system, (c) personality, (d) social system, and (e) cultural system. . . . Second, the sociologist can provide an historical and cross-cultural perspective, enabling the medical student to relate developments in medicine and the organization of medical care to other major areas of human concern such as government, religion and the arts. Third, the conception of alternative responses to illness is important. . . . Finally, the behavioral sciences can contribute significantly to an understanding of such major life experiences in the human life cycle as pregnancy, child birth, infancy, and death. The physician's experiences will be more complete and effective when he can relate his knowledge of biological process to pertinent social, cultural, and personality factors.[25]

Currently, most sociological teaching in schools of public health covers such topics as social and cultural factors in health and disease, the structure and function of health organizations, community organization and process, public opinion and communication, individual and group decision-making processes, social stratification and social change. Most of these courses attempt to introduce this sociological content in the context of current public health problems and practices. The emphasis varies from the highly applied curriculum of the School of Public

Health at the University of California, Los Angeles, whose objective is "to communicate basic principles of organization, administration, and management, with particular application to the contemporary and future problems and practices of public health agencies at state and metropolitan levels,"[26] to the more generalized approach of the Harvard University School of Public Health, which allows students to build up a social science sequence. An interesting aspect of the Harvard program is the mixing of public health and graduate anthropology and sociology students in a single course on "Health and Illness in Cross-Cultural Perspective." Paul reports that "members of the one group are repeatedly intrigued and informed by the unexpected comments coming from the other group."[27]

At the present time, there is little agreement or sharing of ideas concerning what social science concepts and techniques should be taught at schools of public health, and how. The growth of social science courses in these schools has been largely fortuitous and haphazard. There has been little time for the planning, development, and testing of course materials. As the relationship between sociology and public health matures, however, the current emphasis upon a rather general orientation and the inculcation of an accepting attitude must give way to a more solid content of sociological theory and facts related to significant aspects of the health sciences as well as to practical health problems. As is true for all curricula development, however, careful research and evaluation are sorely needed on both content and method of teaching sociology, or any of the social sciences, in the field of public health or any other area of medical education.

At the present time, medical sociology does not as a rule occupy a prominent place in the curricula of traditional academic departments of sociology. Such courses are beginning to appear as graduate seminars and, undoubtedly, will soon find their way into undergraduate education. A strong impetus in this direction will come from the predoctoral and postdoctoral training programs in social science recently established by the National Institute of Mental Health. Aside from these specialized training programs, however, the future development of acceptable courses in medical sociology as part of the regular course offering of academic departments of sociology will probably depend upon the ability of medical sociologists to produce an integrated framework of social theory and health subject matter.

Service Activities

The cultural, social, and psychological aspects of public health practice are receiving increasing attention in the planning and operation of service programs. Many public health programs are failing to achieve their objectives, not because of a lack of medical knowledge but rather as a result of public ignorance, apathy, or resistance. Some of these problems can be overcome through greater awareness of and attention to social factors. For example, large segments, if not the major proportion, of potential clients of public health services in many large urban areas are members of minority groups such as Negroes and Puerto Ricans, and yet little use is being made of the large body of social science knowledge on the attitudes and behavior of these groups. The question arises, however, of the extent to which social scientists could and should become directly involved in applying such knowledge to the actual carrying out of service programs.

This is not a new problem for the social sciences. It has arisen time and again in connection with social action programs aimed at a wide variety of social problems. The issue, however, takes on a somewhat different tone when the problem area already has its prescribed professional workers, and the question becomes one of the extent to which social scientists should or should not assume the working role of the professional in the service field.

As we said earlier, very few sociologists now serve as public health practitioners or even assume part-time service functions. Sociologists, it would seem, when faced with a practical, operational problem, are best at asking questions, somewhat less good at finding answers to these questions, and worse at doing something with the answers. In very few instances have sociologists taken an active role in program operation and when they have participated, it has usually not been as sociologist, but as administrator.

Perhaps this is as it should be, since the sociologist is currently not trained in public health and finds his greatest utility as a consultant on special aspects of public health programs. Some observers have argued that it is important for the protection of the sociologist's status that his role be divorced from the operational aspects of public health programs. If he is to function effectively as a scientist, he should avoid service responsibilities. In order to maintain his identification as a social scientist, he should not permit himself to become involved in the daily operations of public health practice.

In an insightful analysis of social action in the area of population control, Berelson documents a common experience of many social scientists entering an applied professional field—the movement away from social research for the sake of increased knowledge to social research as an aid to action and even participation in the action itself.

> In summary, then, my brief tour of duty so far has led me to some conclusions that do not ordinarily characterize the social researcher in his professional stance. I have moved from initial concern with basic research studies to concern with applied field campaigns or natural experiments, with research coming in primarily as evaluator of outcome. I have moved from concern with motivation to concern for implementation: organization, administration, recruitment, training for programs of family planning. I have moved from an academic approach to what might be called, in the best sense, a professional one. And as a corollary, I have moved from concern with communication research to concern with communication itself.[28]

There can be little doubt that Berelson's changing concerns reflect a natural response to the very real pressures and needs of an action program aimed at the alleviation of an important health problem. But the basic question still remains—is this the proper function, or perhaps more relevant, the most profitable use of the trained social scientist? Certainly the social scientist who wishes to try his hand at "applied field campaigns," "implementation," and "communication itself" should be encouraged, but in so doing it must be clear that he is no longer functioning as a "social scientist"—and it would be a mistake for public health administrators or program developers to assume that the social scientists they employ would carry out such tasks, unless, of course, this had been clearly specified in advance. A failure on the part of a social scientist undertaking such an assignment is not so much an indictment of the state of social science knowledge as it is a reflection of the social scientist's inability to mount a successful action campaign.

To the extent that sociologists wish to limit their primary role to research and consultation, there is much to be said for this kind of objective detachment. But there is an increasing demand for the kind of public health practitioner who knows how to work with community groups, who is aware of the complex processes of public opinion and individual behavior, and who can apply the sociological principles of communication and propaganda. Such a practicing social scientist could bring to public health a new approach to public health education and could take an active part in the planning, development, and operation of a wide variety of public health programs. Despite considerable knowledge about prevention and treatment, the public health problem for many diseases is how to get people to take advantage of this knowledge. Increasingly, the management of illness is becoming a social and behavioral, as well as a medical, problem. Furthermore, the operation of service programs involves not only these external relationships with the public, but internal relationships, interaction, and communication among staff members—a form of administrative science that also has its roots in social science principles and concepts.

Thus there are areas in public health where a well-trained sociologist could assume a service function as a social science practitioner. To be sure, he would need additional training in the technical aspects of public health practice, but his social science background should serve him to advantage in securing community support for public health programs, organizing groups for public health education, formulating internal personnel policies, operating rehabilitation or recreational programs, planning and developing mass detection programs, introducing new public health technologies in underdeveloped areas, and so forth. The field of sociology has already produced operating personnel for such applied professions as social work, marriage and family counseling, business administration, and criminology and corrections. With additional training in public health administration, sociologists should find a fertile field for the application of their knowledge and skills in public health practice.

This is particularly true of those health problems that are also social problems, such as alcoholism, venereal disease, mental illness, and narcotics addiction. The sociologist can help plan a program that will meet the particular social expectations and psychological needs of the individuals affected. As a student of social change, he is also in a good position to anticipate and plan for changing public health needs in the face of changing social conditions.

In a guide developed by the social science staff of the California State Department of Health, the following social components of program operation are identified.

1. Maintaining a public health program that recognizes and deals directly or indirectly with concomitant social problems.
2. Carrying out policies and procedures in health department programs which consider basic needs of children and adults as well as individual and group differences, including staff and community education around these concepts.
3. Helping individuals and groups served by the Health Department to use existing services, within or outside the Health Department, which best meet their health, social, and emotional problems.
4. Bringing to the attention of the community the need for modification and extension of services and programs and reaching an understanding with agencies as to types of referrals and exchange of information that would be mutually helpful.[29]

In carrying out these service functions, the sociologist would contribute his specialized knowledge and skills concerning social and psychological aspects of public health practice as a working member of the overall public health team. In each case, he would be expected to make specific recommendations for action, to help decide how, when, and where a public health program should be established, and then to participate actively in the operation of that program.

In addition to this direct service function, sociologists can make an indirect service contribution in the more established role of consultant to operating programs. Such consultation usually involves only short-term and relatively shallow involvement of the sociologist in actual programs. He may visit and observe the program in operation, interview both the public health workers and the individuals or groups they are dealing with, examine existing records and available data, participate briefly in the service program, and on the basis of this first-hand experience make recommendations which take into account the sociological aspects of the public health problem. Several illuminating case studies of social science consultation in connection with the conduct of environmental health programs in a large metropolitan health department deal with the social, cultural, and behavioral components of such problems as water pollution, air pollution, food market inspection, and rat control. These case studies dramatically illustrate the kind of service a social scientist can offer in helping the public health professional meet the everyday problems of public health work.[30]

To some extent, a certain amount of difficulty will be created by differing definitions, and hence incongruous expectations, of what constitutes research or service on the part of the public health professional and the sociologist. What the public health worker perceives as a research activity may strike the sociologist as being rather straightforward service, and, vice versa, a sociologist may be performing what he considers a service function but looks like research to the public health practitioner. Similarly, both groups may have conflicting definitions of what constitutes consultation. A public health worker may often think he is involving the social scientist in a research project, while the social scientist sees his role as being limited to consultation. This selective labeling often creates a misleading image of the social sciences and social science activities, both for the public health personnel and for the social scientists themselves. Thus even the social science disciplines may present an inaccurate professional image.

In discussing the strategy of socio-medical research in relation to service functions, Williams indicates several advantages that can accrue to research conducted in the context of an operating problem. Such service involvement not only helps to "pay the freight" of the sociologist and to validate his role in the eyes of the practicing professional, it also has direct strategic importance in familiarizing the sociologist with the layman's hypotheses and in helping to close the gap between theory and reality.[31] Gouldner describes the importance of this function of service research as follows:

> . . . The latent function of such tests, however, is to document the inadequacy and breakdown of lay hypotheses, thus enlarging the area of intellectual discretion allowable to applied social scientists, and easing their introduction of independent variables that are novel to laymen.[32]

Williams also points out that the sociologist in an applied field such as public health must recognize the requirements of service activities even though he is least well prepared for them. He warns against the sociologist assuming any direct treatment functions, however, and stresses the consultative role in helping the practitioners to define their problems more clearly and systematically. In the case of public health, he does perceive a possible direct service contribution of sociologists in community organization and development, including the utilization of services, but advises additional formal and in-service training involving some "secondary professionalization" in public health.

We have already noted, in the previous chapters, the many areas of sociological theory and method that impinge upon public health activities. The potential contribution of social research to the planning and development of a wide range of public health programs is clear. The question now is whether or not sociologists should venture beyond their research and consultant status into public health practice. At present, the answer to this question depends a great deal upon the personal inclinations of the individual sociologist. Certainly a tremendous opportunity is available to those sociologists who wish to become practitioners. However, it is important to point out that the assumption of such a service role will probably require the relinquishing of one's primary identification as a social scientist. Just as a biostatistician or engineer, and to some extent a physician, who joins a health agency and assumes responsibility for operating a public health program comes to think of himself as a public health professional, so must the sociologist who becomes actively engaged in public health practice give up his rather limited commitment to the public health field and form new group allegiances. This shift will undoubtedly require additional graduate training in public health, and several schools of public health now offer graduate degrees in public health to sociologically trained students.

Preparation for Work in Public Health

Few, if any, sociologists in the field of public health today prepared themselves specifically for work in this area. A good background in the behavioral sciences, both content and methods, and research experience have gone a long way. However, it is probable that a more custom-made course of training will be offered in the near future.

The sociologist who is planning to enter the public health field needs first and foremost a sound training in basic social science theory and methods, including social psychology and cultural anthropology. With this background of basic knowledge, he can then take more advanced courses in specific areas such as public opinion and communication, community organization, and group dynamics. Courses in social problems such as the aged, mental illness, race relations, and population would have relevance for many current public health problems. Basic courses should also be taken in economics and political science, with emphasis upon problems of the cost of medical care and program administration.

Also important, in addition to a sound theoretical background, is training in research methods and statistics, including demography and ecology. The sociologist who brings to public health the research skills involved in formulating a research design, in sample selection, in questionnaire construction, and in the analysis of data will find a ready market for his abilities. Advanced training in statistics, including biostatistics, is a very real advantage.

Respondents to the Health Information Foundation survey of medical sociologists supported this need for a sound theoretical and methodological background before entering the applied field. In general, they believed that a medical sociologist should be, first of all, a good sociologist. To achieve this, they recommended a liberal arts background which would provide a sound theoretical base in social science. Graduate work should be on a broad and integrated interdisciplinary base, including anthropology, psychology, and social psychology, and should include extensive training in research methods and statistics.[33]

Postgraduate training might include a year of study in a school of public health. Several of the schools of public health offer special training programs for behavioral scientists interested in public health, administrative medicine, or medical care. Such postgraduate training will give the sociologist a valuable background in public health practice, public health education, epidemiology, biostatistics, medical economics, and administrative medicine. Many of these programs offer predoctoral fellowships for behavioral scientists. In exceptional cases, depending upon the type of public health work envisioned, it might be advantageous for the student majoring in sociology to consider matriculating for a medical degree before undertaking advanced training in public health. Stanford University, under a grant from Russell Sage Foundation, has designed a distinctive program known as the Stanford Program in Medicine and the Behavioral Sciences. The objectives of this program include: systematic incorporation of behavioral concepts and methods into the medical curriculum, encouragement of some medical students to undertake specialized work in social science while pursuing the M.D. degree, provision for more adequate preparation of social scientists who intend to specialize in the field of health, encouragement of joint medical-behavioral science research, and preparation of teaching materials to be used in interdisciplinary education. Russell Sage Foundation has also supported social science training programs at the Schools of Public Health at Harvard and the University of California in Berkeley.

Research experience may be obtained in a variety of ways. Social research on social problems is similar enough to research in the field of public health to permit high transferability of training. Public health research experience can be obtained by working for any of the numerous health projects being conducted by universities or by voluntary or public health agencies. The Inventory of Research of the Health Information Foundation lists more than 350 such agencies currently conducting research programs on the social or economic aspects of health.

Much of the sociologist's specialized training in public health can be secured from intensive reading while on the job. The sociologist entering public health today is not expected to know the public health field—only to be willing to make the effort to learn. For a sociologist willing to make this effort, the field of public health offers many exciting opportunities in research, teaching, and service.

NOTES TO CHAPTER VII

1. Bloom, Samuel W., A. Wessen, R. Straus, G. Reader, and J. Myers, "The Sociologist as a Medical Educator: A Discussion," *American Sociological Review*, vol. 25, February, 1960, pp. 96–101.
2. Wellin, Edward, *Uses of the Behavioral (Social) Sciences in Public Health*. Prepared under contract and submitted to the National Institute of Mental Health, July, 1961. Mimeographed.
3. *Report of the Surgeon General to Ad Hoc Committee on Mental Health Activities*. U.S. Public Health Service, Washington, August, 1962. Mimeographed.
4. Hawkins, Norman G., *Medical Sociology*. Charles C Thomas, Springfield, Ill., 1958, pp. 112–113.
5. Anderson, Odin W., and Milvoy S. Seacat, *An Analysis of Personnel in Medical Sociology*. Health Information Foundation, Research Series 21, New York, 1962.
6. Williams, Richard H., "The Strategy of Socio-Medical Research" in Freeman, Howard, Sol Levine, and Leo G. Reeder, editors, *The Handbook of Medical Sociology*. Prentice-Hall, Inc., Englewood Cliffs, N. J., 1963, p. 434.
7. James, George, "Research by Local Health Departments—Problems, Methods, Results," *American Journal of Public Health*, vol. 48, March, 1958, p. 353.
8. Boek, Walter E., *An Introduction to a Long-Range Research Program in Public Health*. New York State Department of Health, Albany, N. Y., January 30, 1953.
9. Williams, Richard H., *op. cit.*, p. 432.
10. Anderson, Odin W., and Milvoy S. Seacat, *The Behavioral Scientists and Research in the Health Field*. Health Information Foundation, Research Series 1, New York, 1957.
11. Anderson, Odin W., and Milvoy S. Seacat, *op. cit.*, 1962, p. 4. (See note 5.)
12. Wellin, Edward, and Milvoy S. Seacat, "Social Science in the Health Field: A Review of Research (1954–1959)," *American Journal of Public Health*, vol. 52, September, 1962, pp. 1465–1472.
13. Bloom, Samuel W., and others, *op. cit.*, p. 97.
14. Troupin, James L., "Schools of Public Health in the United States and Canada: 1959–1960," *American Journal of Public Health*, vol. 50, November, 1960, pp. 1–22.
15. Straus, Robert, "The Nature and Status of Medical Sociology," *American Sociological Review*, vol. 22, April, 1957, pp. 200–204.
16. Buck, Rodger L., "Behavioral Scientists in Schools of Medicine," *Journal of Health and Human Behavior*, vol. 2, Spring, 1961, pp. 59–64.

17. Anderson, Odin W., and Milvoy S. Seacat, *op. cit.*, 1962, p. 4.
18. Buck, Rodger L., *op. cit.*, p. 63.
19. Paul, Benjamin D., "Teaching Cultural Anthropology in Schools of Public Health" in Mandelbaum, David G., and others, editors, *The Teaching of Anthropology*. In press.
20. Jaco, E. Gartly, "Problems and Practices of the Social Sciences in Medical Education," *Journal of Health and Human Behavior*, vol. 1, Spring, 1960, pp. 29–34.
21. Straus, Robert, "A Department of Behavioral Science," *Journal of Medical Education*, vol. 34, July, 1959, p. 666.
22. Paul, Benjamin D., *op. cit.*
23. Troupin, James L., *op. cit.*, p. 14.
24. Macgregor, Frances Cooke, *Social Science in Nursing*. Russell Sage Foundation, New York, 1960.
25. Bloom, Samuel W., and others, *op. cit.*, pp. 99–100.
26. University of California, Los Angeles, School of Public Health, *A Proposed Curriculum of Graduate Instruction in Public Health Administration*, January, 1961, p. 1. Mimeographed.
27. Paul, Benjamin D., *op. cit.*
28. Berelson, Bernard, "Communication, Communication Research, and Family Planning," *The Emerging Techniques in Population Research*. Proceedings of the 39th Conference of the Milbank Memorial Fund, New York, 1963.
29. California State Department of Health, "Identification of Social Components in Health Department Programs: A Guide Developed by the Social Service Staff," *American Journal of Public Health*, vol. 45, January, 1955, p. 125.
30. *Conference Workbook*. First National Conference on Human Behavior and Environmental Health, Philadelphia, Pennsylvania, January 24–26, 1961. Mimeographed.
31. Williams, Richard H., "The Strategy of Socio-Medical Research" in Freeman, Levine, and Reeder, editors, *op. cit.*, p. 440.
32. Gouldner, Alvin W., "Theoretical Requirements of the Applied Social Science," *American Sociological Review*, vol. 22, February, 1957, p. 95.
33. Anderson, Odin W., and Milvoy S. Seacat, *op. cit.*, 1962, p. 6.

VIII

PATTERNS OF COLLABORATION AND INTERACTION

WHEN THE SOCIOLOGIST leaves the safe and familiar home grounds of the university to enter the field of public health, he faces a new and strange world of different, and perhaps even threatening, values and personalities as well as concepts and methods. He must learn to live in this world because he is there for the explicit purpose of collaborative effort and there can be no valid retreat into independent work. As a professional sociologist, he brings with him specific knowledge and skills and, perhaps just as important, a point of view and approach to health problems which constitute his unique contribution to the kind of interdisciplinary teamwork that characterizes much of public health today.

In appraising the reception given to sociology by public health, it is important to keep in mind the relatively recent development of this relationship. Any early period of collaboration between professional fields is bound to be one of mixed enthusiasm and disappointment. Both sociologist and public health worker are going through a period of adjustment, learning each other's ways of thinking and talking, defining their respective roles and responsibilities, and, mostly, seeking to establish some working relationship that will prove mutually profitable to each of them.

As Goode points out, "No specialty develops inside a profession without antagonism."[1] This is particularly likely to be the case for sociology which has difficulty in defining for itself any precise function or even problem area. About the best a sociologist can do at this stage is to "identify his skill: 'I solve sociological problems.'"[2] In addition, the results of social research are not likely to be characterized by the impersonality of medical research and may actually threaten the value system or customary mode of behavior of the public health practitioner.

A sociologist entering the field of public health faces collaborative problems on a number of different levels and with a number of different occupational groups. First, he is subject to the ordinary strains of any interdisciplinary effort, aggravated perhaps by the fact that the scientific background of his collaborators is likely to be in the basic biological sciences of medicine, with their greater emphasis upon the experimental method of the laboratory. Second, he is subject to the perhaps even more difficult strains of a researcher-practitioner relationship. The field of public health is largely an applied field with a major emphasis upon the solution of practical problems, while sociology is a basic science with an orientation toward seeking knowledge without particular regard for its practicality. Thus the sociologist in the field of public health has a double handicap when it comes to establishing working relationships with public health practitioners. Not only does he have the well-known strains of any research person who attempts to study an operating program—differences in value-orientations, in goals, in personality, in methods of thought and work; he is also subject to a disciplinary strain between social science and medical science. The social scientist is a stranger, as well as a research worker who may interfere with the conduct of a service activity.

In general, the public health sociologist must maintain interpersonal working relationships with three main groups of individuals: (1) the public health practitioner charged with the administrative responsibility of operating health programs; (2) the public health research worker, engaged in either (a) basic research or (b) applied research; and (3) the sociologist who is either (a) also in the field of public health, or (b) not in the field of public health. Each of these groups presents somewhat different problems in collaboration, with group 1 probably creating the most difficulty by demanding answers to operational problems quite foreign to the sociologist untrained in public health, followed by group 2a, where differences will center largely on the adequacy of the sociologist's definition and measurement of social concepts, and group 2b, where the formulation of the research problem and the interpretation of findings as recommendations for action may create the greatest obstacles to collaboration. Group 3, consisting of other sociologists, will find 3a providing the most rewarding and stimulating opportunities for sharing experiences, while 3b will often constitute an uncertain reference group whose approval or disapproval will continue to be important to the public health sociologist.

A recent report of Russell Sage Foundation presents an informative analysis of problems in collaboration between social scientists and practitioners, based upon reports from 65 social scientists engaged in Russell Sage Foundation-supported projects in the health and other applied fields. According to the Foundation's *Annual Report, 1958–1959*, these problems may be divided into three major categories:

1. Differing cultural backgrounds which affect language, values, goals, and perceptions;
2. Low-status work within a rigid, status-conscious institutional setting;
3. Differing conceptions of self and expectations of others.

This Report constitutes the only systematic description available of problems in collaboration between social scientists and practitioners and is worth quoting in some detail:

> Cultural differences are the source of many problems in collaborative efforts. When people from widely differing cultural backgrounds are put into situations requiring cooperation in a joint undertaking . . . they will have trouble in understanding one another, in agreeing on the facts of the situation, and on the important goals to which effort should be directed. . . . All subgroups of a society tend to develop their own ways of perceiving and conceptualizing the "facts" of their concerns; their own particular goals and scales of values; their own language, meaningful to them but jargon to the outsider; and their own body of technology by which they operate on the objects of their special concerns. . . .
>
> A second group of problems mentioned by our social scientists can be identified as those derived from the nature of the setting in which they work and from the position or status they occupy in that setting. A rather rigid bureaucratic, authoritarian, status-conscious institutional situation is not an easy setting for a representative of a new,

relatively unknown, and low-status science to test and demonstrate the relevance and utility of his discipline. . . .

A large third group of problems stems from the lack of clarity in, and the incongruities of, conceptions of self and expectations of others when social scientists and professional practitioners interact. These problems are most acute, of course, in the early phase of collaborative undertakings. Social scientists frequently suffer from the misapprehension that the professions to which they go know nothing about social science and, consequently, they begin to perform as missionaries and propagandists with predictable results. . . .[3]

These three groups of problems distributed themselves in almost equal proportions: 36 per cent, type 1; 26 per cent, type 2; and 36 per cent, type 3. Problems related to the satisfactory definition of one's role and the development of congruent expectations were mentioned most often by social scientists working in the health field, 63 per cent, while only 6 per cent described problems involving cultural differences of values or goals. This finding was quite the opposite for the fields of law, social work, and theology.

Despite these problems of collaboration, the Russell Sage Foundation Report concludes that an overwhelming majority of Foundation projects resulted in highly productive undertakings.

The Health Information Foundation survey of behavioral scientists working in the health field found that, while only a small minority of the professional health personnel understood the value of the behavioral sciences in the health field, a much larger proportion were described as willing to cooperate. It is reassuring to note that public health personnel were rated highest of all the health professions both in understanding and in cooperation. The authors of the study go on to say:

For a behavioral scientist, it makes no sense to "blame" physicians for being uncooperative or nurses for not "understanding the role of behavioral science" and so on. Such reactions—real or imagined—are part of the objective situations with which behavioral scientists have to work, and should be evaluated as such. Imaginative strategy and tactics of a very high order are called for. In fact, specific training may be less necessary than emphasis on general theoretical considerations, skills in analyzing the components of problems and the groups involved, general training in technique of research and

Cultural Differences

consultation, and preparation in adapting spoken and written English to audiences other than behavioral scientists.[4]

Let us look for a moment at the basic differences in the values and assumptions of the social scientist and the public health practitioner, especially as these are reflected in differing objectives or goals. One way of examining these differences is in terms of the prejudices and misperceptions that interfere with communication and collaboration between the social scientist and the practicing professional. As in the case of most instances of prejudice, individual differences succumb to group stereotypes. The practitioner may at times think of the social scientist in such negative stereotypes as a rather fuzzy-minded, impractical, verbose, undisciplined interloper. The social scientist, on his part, may form a stereotype of the practitioner as a narrow-minded, uncreative, anti-intellectual, biased job-holder. Like most stereotypes, these collective images reflect the influence of personality and value systems upon the social perception of the half-truths of reality.

Neither group likes to have its basic assumptions challenged. The public health practitioner does not like to be asked such fundamental questions as "What right do you have to urge people to follow what you believe are good health habits, for instance, eating different foods, taking preventive vaccinations, not bathing in polluted waters?" As in virtually all professional fields, there is a whole folklore of accepted beliefs and practices. The public health educator, for the most part, still continues to believe in the efficacy of printed pamphlets and booklets. The nutritionist still tends to think that people can be told what to eat. Forcing these practitioners into a probing self-examination of their "taken for granted" beliefs and practices can be painful and annoying.

On the other hand, the social scientist does not like to have his vaguely defined and beloved concepts constantly challenged. He likes to believe that his field of knowledge is based upon scientifically proved facts. He resists, also, the probing self-examination into long-held, cherished theories and generalizations.

These differing expectations and definitions of the situation set the stage for defensive reactions. Otherwise reasonable individuals assume the role of representatives of their special field of interest and fight for the good name and reputation of their discipline. All of the mechanisms of prejudice are called into play. Ethnocentrism replaces objective, individual judgment.

And, as is usual with prejudice, propaganda is less effective than personal interaction. Professional group identification and disciplinary allegiance must give way to individual communication and interaction. Both the social scientist and public health practitioner must live and work together as members of a team tackling a common problem. With the emphasis on a specific, shared task, individuals do not feel the same need to defend their status and role positions. Thus it is probably undesirable for either group to insist upon a clear-cut definition that underscores the respective disciplinary memberships.

Role and Status Problems

We have already noted in Chapter VII the general problem of defining the sociologist's function and position in the public health organization. It is much too early in the development of working relationships between sociologists and public health personnel to attempt to formulate any standardized definition of job function or to describe the most desirable status position or pattern of role relationship. At present, each sociologist in each organization needs to develop his own "modus vivendi." At this stage, we can only point out some of the problems that have arisen in regard to the sociologist's role and status in health organizations.

Perhaps the most important problem the sociologist in public health has to face is that of role identification. The sociologist working in a public health agency or even a school of public health or medicine is likely to find himself isolated from his sociological colleagues. Adair has characterized him as having a "lonely reference group." In many senses of the word, he becomes a "marginal" man. He is not fully accepted by the public health profession, and he may be partly rejected by his own social science discipline. Both tend to view his work with skepticism. In very few cases can he fully please both groups. In this marginal position he may find it difficult to establish any clear-cut role relationship with either group, and he may be tempted to develop some group identification of his own, such as medical sociologist.

To the extent that this type of specialized group membership interferes with the medical sociologist's identity as sociologist, it would also tend to destroy his unique contribution as a sociologist. If sociology as a discipline has any meaningful relationship to public health, it must come from the basic concepts, theories, and methods of sociology. While sociologists in public health may perform many useful functions and work on a wide variety of health problems, they will make their most outstanding contribution as sociologists by adhering closely to the basic content and method of their parent discipline. There is little to be served by the sociologist's becoming another kind of public health technician.

Freeman, Levine, and Reeder point out some of the dangers inherent in the current tendency of many sociologists in the health field to weaken their professional identification in order to attain easier acceptance by the medical practitioner. Foremost among these dangers is the possibility that medical sociology may develop as a "guild-like" structure rather than a scholarly discipline. They warn against "the subjugation of sociologists into action roles" and strongly advise the sociologist in the health field to protect his professional identity and autonomy as a social scientist.[5]

To help overcome the isolation of the lone sociologist in a public health setting and to increase the probability of his preserving his professional identity as a sociologist, Williams recommends a continuing relationship between the sociologist and some academic group, perhaps even a joint university appointment wherever possible. He also suggests bringing in outside sociologists as consultants and encouraging the sociologist to attend professional meetings.[6] There is a real danger, however, that this natural desire to maintain professional relationships with one's discipline may be misinterpreted by public health practitioners as representing a lack of commitment to public health on the part of the sociologist.

The importance of status factors in the success or failure of the sociologist entering a public health organization is emphasized by the Russell Sage Foundation Report on the basis of its survey. The social scientist cannot hope for successful collaboration with public health professionals unless he is given high enough status to warrant their acceptance and respect. As summarized in the *Annual Report, 1958–1959*, of Russell Sage Foundation:

> Running throughout the problems that derive from situational structure are the ubiquitous problems of status differentials. Professions like theology, medicine, and law are endowed with the pride of an ancient and honorable past, rich in tradition and lustrous in achievement. Their present positions are weighty and respected. One whose own status is based on a new, relatively untried field is obviously disadvantaged in dealing with members of such professions.... Different and somewhat more difficult types of status problems are encountered when dealing with professional groups who themselves occupy somewhat weak or uncertain status positions.[7]

In addition to being given a high enough position in the status hierarchy to permit his voice to be heard, the sociologist should be placed whenever possible in a staff position where he can report directly to the head of the health agency. As Williams points out, the sociologist performs a general function related to the overall mission of the agency and locating him in one subdivision or bureau not only creates a danger of identification with one segment of the total organization but also places a non-social scientist as intermediary between him and the top administration, often leading to distortion and frustration.

As time goes on, there is little doubt that the sociologists in public health, like the statisticians, bacteriologists, and sanitary engineers before them, will find their accepted place in public health work. To some extent, this will mean loosening their sociological affiliations and forming new ties with public health organizations and professional activities. It will mean the growth of a new reference group from the field of public health. Until this mature stage of development is reached, however, we must continue to expect growing pains and a certain amount of sibling rivalry and maternal dependence.

Collaboration in an Applied Setting

Perhaps the greatest difference in general point of view between sociologist and public health practitioner concerns the relative emphasis to be placed upon applied or basic research, upon action or understanding, upon practice or theory. Public health itself is an applied science, and when it turns to sociology, it is for help in making its operating programs more effective. It is understandable, therefore, that much of the current controversy over the place of sociology in the field of public health concerns the issue of basic versus applied science.

The fundamental nature of this difference in orientation between the sociologist as scientist and researcher and the public health professional as practitioner and administrator is stressed by Foster as a major problem in collaboration between social science and public health.

> The work of this kind of (social) scientist is exploratory; he wants to find out, to know; he wants to order knowledge in meaningful patterns; he wants to build theory. He is not immediately concerned, as a scientist, with the goodness or badness of his discoveries, nor with their immediate practical utilization. The practice of public health, on the other hand, is a profession . . . it is a directly applied venture. The existence of a public health organization means that health problems have been defined, that it has been deemed desirable to solve these problems, and that a bureaucracy has been created to work toward the solution of these problems. . . . In other words, an academic discipline stresses theoretical research, while a profession stresses goal-directed practice. The two aims are by no means mutually exclusive, but they are different. . . . Not only are the aims of disciplines and professions distinct, but the ego-satisfying criteria are also different. Public health personnel feel gratified when they know they have raised the level of health in their jurisdiction through their efforts, and that this success is recognized by their colleagues. Behavioral scientists feel gratified when they feel they have made new contributions to basic science, and when these contributions are acknowledged by their colleagues.[8]

Without engaging in a fruitless debate over the relative differences and merits of applied versus basic science, we would like to express our conviction that there is need and the opportunity for both in the field of public health. The social epidemiology of the chronic diseases, with its strong accent on social stress and "way of life" variables, calls for the best theory and method of "pure" social science, while the changing of individual and community attitudes and behavior regarding health and illness will require sophisticated "social engineering." However, the sociologist who enters the field of public health via an operating agency, such as a public or voluntary health organization, or a hospital, must be prepared, just as the physiologist or biologist before him, to forgo some of his disciplinary purity in a coordinated attack upon some specific public health problem. Many of the current problems of collaboration hinge upon this willingness to see oneself as a working member of a public health team as well as a professional sociologist.

The need for the knowledge-oriented sociologist and the action-oriented public health worker to recognize and accept each other's point of view is emphasized by Anderson and Gordon in an analysis of social research in the health field.

> A lack of understanding has often existed between health personnel and social scientists, limiting the effectiveness of social research. Health personnel have frequently judged social research in terms of its immediate usefulness to the solution of their problems. . . . The social scientist, on the other hand, has often viewed the problems of health personnel as of little moment. Consequently, he has often restated problems in terms which are important to social scientists but which are relatively useless from the health association's standpoint. . . . It is unrealistic for the social scientist to submerge the needs of health personnel to the needs of social science. An effective approach to social research incorporates existing social theory and data and attempts to add to that knowledge in terms of an immediate problem.[9]

To some extent, the division between basic and applied science is a matter of arbitrary definition. In the real world of public health practice, however, this separation is likely to become a matter of heated controversy. The public health worker is faced with practical problems that demand immediate decisions, if not solutions, based upon whatever facts are available, regardless of their adequacy. The social scientist, on the other hand, is reluctant to make recommendations for action based upon his findings unless he feels that these are validly supported by the data. The social scientist is also more likely to feel that research which investigates basic hypotheses will, in the long run, prove most practical, while the public health practitioner appears less interested in more widespread future gains at the expense of an immediate answer to the problem he is facing at the moment.

If it were not for limited resources of time, budget, and personnel, the solution would probably be one of a division of labor, with different individuals working on both basic and applied research. However, work in any operating agency will always require an assignment of priorities, and an ever-present danger lies in the social scientist being swallowed by the dozens of immediate "putting-out-of-fire" jobs that arise each day. While the social scientist must avoid becoming a "chore boy," he must also be willing on occasion to lay aside his concern with more basic issues to pitch in on operating problems, in order to avoid the public health administrator's exasperated plea, "Why can't he forget his professional identification long enough to get the job done?" The sociologist must recognize that public health activity will proceed anyway and that action must often be taken on the basis of the best available knowledge without stopping to do research. Simon emphasizes the goal of "satisficing" in applied research, or seeking a course of action that is "good enough." He suggests the idea of "bounded rationality" as determining how a theoretical model might be applied to actual behavior. "Art," in this sense, might be viewed as the science of practitioner behavior.[10]

Probably one of the most productive ways for the social scientist to look at applied research in public health is to recognize that applied research has its own "basic theory." Administration is the science of decision-making. Almost any operating problem can be broken down into a complex of social factors affecting the administrative decision. With experience the social researcher will be able to detect factors of relevance to basic social science in almost any practical problem, no matter how trivial it may appear at first. It is essential, however, in analyzing these basic factors, that the social researcher keep in mind the practical problem at hand and remember that the reason for seeking a more basic formulation of the problem is not only to increase its sociological significance but also to permit the possibility of arriving at an answer that has relevance for the immediate problem and *for others of a similar class.*

To some degree, this difference in goal-orientation of the social researcher and the public health practitioner reflects a much deeper conflict in a whole mode of thought—what might be called conceptual versus operational thinking. Coming from an academic setting, the social scientist may be surprised at the difficulty he sometimes encounters among practitioners in communication on a more general level of abstraction. Many practitioners do not feel at home with complex concepts and abstract thoughts. The sociologist is likely to find that most operational ideas are not expressed with great generality and that little attempt is made to relate specific problems to larger issues. The practitioner, on the other hand, may find the social scientist's attempts to state practical problems in terms of more general concepts an annoying and at times an unrealistic approach. The practitioner is likely to want to talk about clinical cases while the social scientist will want to generalize.

The practitioner must gradually learn to see within the specific, the more general implications. The social scientist, on his part, must be willing to leave the safety of the general or abstract and to venture into the more treacherous waters of specific cases. He must also learn to respect the importance of actual clinical problems and not feel that saving "one fallen sparrow" is less worthwhile than a treatise on saving sparrows in general.

An excellent picture of some of the mutual frustrations of the social scientist and the public health practitioner can be secured from the findings of a study on the utilization of research findings in an operational setting. According to the practitioner, some of the major sources of friction are due to the following failings of the social researcher:

1. Research workers are woefully deficient in professional knowledge.
2. Research workers seem consistently to ignore the question posed by the agency and to go off on methodological tangents.
3. Research workers camouflage their reports in technical jargon.

4. Research workers fail to involve practitioners in the crucial planning and recommendation stages.

While, according to the researcher:

1. Practitioners and administrators are woefully deficient in knowledge of research methodology and are particularly deficient in knowing how to pose a question so that meaningful research can be carried out.
2. Practitioners and administrators are not interested in furthering knowledge in the field. They want easy formulas for quick action.
3. Practitioners and administrators are antiscientific. They prefer to operate on dogma rather than research.
4. Practitioners and administrators want all research to prove their biases, not to test propositions. In short, they want to see only favorable findings.
5. Practitioners and administrators don't read research reports because it would involve careful study and hard thinking.[11]

Any sociologist who has had actual experience working for an operating health agency will recognize the validity of many of these accusations and counter-accusations. There is more than an element of truth in both sides of the controversy, and it should be evident that what is called for is a mature recognition of opposing needs and points of view, with a greater emphasis upon the many ways in which basic and applied research can advance each other.

This way of meeting the problems of applied versus basic research is also emphasized by Herring in the *Annual Report, 1959–1960,* of the Social Science Research Council.

> Consider the arguments over the merits and priorities of basic versus applied research. The research scholar points out that the choice of subject matter is best determined not by the urgencies of public policy or social need but by what will best yield knowledge that can be verified by the use of rigorous method and theory. The rejoinder is that the research that is worthwhile is the kind that can be utilized in dealing with social problems. . . . While the distinctions between basic and applied research are valid, the problem is not one of choosing between such alternatives. The opportunities today are such that social scientists can largely follow their own inclinations insofar as a policy of orientation or a more theoretical approach is concerned. . . . The real problems of the scientists or

scholar are at the working level of finding the theories or methods for analyzing questions of public policy in a constructive fashion, or identifying the research approach that will yield fundamental knowledge regardless of whether the subject may seem trivial or esoteric to the layman.[12]

A recent conference on "Social Research in Health and Welfare Agencies" brought together social research workers and administrators to discuss mutual problems of collaboration. The conflicts aired at this conference were very real ones, reflecting honest differences of opinion concerning the rights and obligations of social scientists in health and welfare agencies. The administrators attending this meeting tended to feel that the salary an administrator paid the social scientist entitled the administrator to define the problems to be studied, and to decide how the findings should be applied. The social scientists, in turn, insisted that their professional integrity demanded that they exercise a certain amount of control over what was studied and how the findings were used. The wide range of conflicting opinions expressed by social researchers and administrators at this meeting makes it obvious, as one participant remarked, that, "Researchers and administrators both would be wise to be sure in their own minds of what they expect their reciprocal responsibilities to be, and to be sure that they share the same expectations."[13]

Perhaps what we are witnessing today are the birth pains of a new profession—the applied social scientist or behavioral science practitioner. This developing profession of "social engineering" naturally faces many new problems of role and status, scientific objectivity, collaboration, and communication. Applied science has attained a highly respected position in such fields as engineering and agriculture, and what seems to be happening today is the growth of an applied social science in the field of public health and medicine. An insightful analysis by Gouldner points out some of the major theoretical requirements of such an applied field of social science. Those that are most relevant to the present discussion include:

1. Applied social science is characterized by an orientation to the values of laymen, as well as of scientists. These lay values, ex-

trinsic to science as such, are regarded by the applied social scientist as legitimate points of orientation for his professional and scientific work.

2. Applied social scientists are more likely to use laymen as a reference group in organizing their professional work, and their work is more likely to occur in the context of, and be influenced by, their relationship with laymen.

3. In dealing with lay "social problems," the applied social scientist is confronting questions for which laymen often believe they have answers. Laymen usually have some explanation or favored hypotheses concerning the source of their problems. However inadequate the applied social scientist may judge these to be, he cannot blithely ignore them.

4. The applied social scientist not only focuses on social problems perceivable to laymen but also requires knowledge to remedy them. Applied social science, therefore, is greatly concerned with facilitating the prediction and production of social and cultural change.

5. The applied social scientist's criteria for assessing the adequacy of an independent variable include predictive potency but go beyond this, adding certain standards not relevant to the pure scientist. For one, the applied social scientist inspects his independent variables to determine the extent to which they are accessible to control.

6. The applied social scientist's interest in unforeseen events is, in important part, a focus on events that laymen find threatening. Stated differently, it is an interest in events over which laymen have lost control and for which, therefore, their need for assistance in regaining it has become manifest.

7. One of the needs of applied social science, therefore, is for the full development of a generalized theory of unanticipated consequences. Consistent, though not identical with this, is a need for a diversity of concepts, varying with the field of application, which direct laymen's attention to patterns of behavior and belief of which he was unaware.[14]

Toward this development of a systematic analysis of the basic structure of an applied social science, we may add the following general considerations:

1. The audience for applied social research findings will be much more limited than for more general research, and the media of

communication are likely to be the restricted memoranda or mimeographed reports rather than articles published in scholarly journals.

2. The applied social scientist will probably face many extraneous pressures that are unrelated to research itself, but reflect the desire to use this research as a vehicle for attaining prestige, building staff, improving public relations, political maneuvering, and the like.

3. The research problems in applied social science usually originate with some operational problem, and may require translation into researchable terms—but the results must then be re-translated into operational terms with specific implications or recommendations for action.

4. Program testing that evaluates the net worth of a whole series of actions or events is more likely to be the objective of applied research than will the testing of separate variables or independent hypotheses. The major objective will be to determine the ability of the program to attain some desired goal rather than to understand *why* it did or did not work.

The foregoing principles and characteristics differentiate the goals and methods of applied research from basic research. To the extent that these factors can be identified and organized, applied research will be able to develop into a systematic approach toward problem-solving. Recognition of the similarities and differences between applied and basic research will do much to remove the conflict between the two and to show how and where they can complement each other. To the sociologist contemplating research in the field of public health, an understanding of these underlying principles of applied research will provide a rational basis for deciding whether one wishes to do this type of research and, if so, what changes one must be ready to accept in terms of objectives and methods. To the public health professional, these characteristics of an applied science should clarify what he can reasonably expect from social research in the field of public health.

Resolution of Conflicts

As reported by the Russell Sage Foundation study, the barriers to collaboration between the social sciences and the practicing professions are complex and not easy to overcome; they require "a very substantial part of the time and energy on both sides . . . even when the parties to the undertaking appeared eager to collaborate fully." The survey found that it was much simpler for their respondents to report problems than to offer solutions. In general, however, five categories of action emerge from the study which appear to offer some promise for improving collaborative relationships.

1. Developing an optimal initial orientation and level of expectation on the part of both the social scientist and the public health practitioner. There should also be a built-in arrangement for periodic reviews and re-definitions.
2. Maximizing mutual assimilation of professional subcultural values, ideologies, technologies, and language. Each party needs to assimilate a working knowledge of the other's field through mutual instruction on a planned basis.
3. Securing an appropriate structural position in the institutional setting for the social scientist. He must be given the usual prerogatives of autonomy in his research with full access to policymakers.
4. Clarification of the roles of the parties to the undertaking. The social scientist must accept responsibility for developing the proper role of social scientist and not pseudo-practitioner.
5. Increasing the interpersonal skills of the participants. While personal qualities, skills, and modes of responding are important, "personality clashes" all too frequently are offered as explanations for difficulties which could be more accurately perceived and more efficiently dealt with as cultural, social-structural, and role-specification problems.[15]

In the development of productive working relationships, there will be a tendency to try to set up a series of "rules of conduct" to govern everyday interaction. It is doubtful that any handbook can cover the dozens of new situations that are bound to rise in the course of an action program. In the long run, certain policy statements may prove more valuable than any specific blueprint for personal conduct. On the basis of our experience, we would like to offer the following four statements as fundamental to a productive working relationship between sociology and public health.

1. *The problem of "needs" has to be viewed from the point of view of social science as well as public health.* The traditional personnel policy of public health has been to employ specialists such as sanitarians, public health nurses, and public health educators, and to direct their work largely into service channels. But as of today, there are few qualified sociologists who are willing to undertake routine service or research functions, important and legitimate as these may be. There is a real danger that, unless work in the public health field can be made to offer gratifications of a professional social science nature, only the "discards" among trained sociologists will be made available to the field. Furthermore, one may seriously question whether either the public health administrator or the sociologist is in a position to define what the *routine* service or research functions of a social scientist should be. There is little gain in employing social scientists who are then assigned the same tasks as the public health worker without social science training.

2. *Any social science program in public health must accept the responsibility of working on problems that are meaningful and useful to public health.* A social scientist who enters the field of public health must do so with a sense of commitment to the needs of public health. It is our conviction that any public health research project that deals with social science concepts can and should make itself understood and useful to the public health practitioner concerned with this problem. Furthermore, when the social scientist's "home" is in an operating health department, he has the further obligation to make recommendations for policy and procedure, even if this requires him "to go beyond his data," as it often will. In addition, the social science program should constantly attempt to be of assistance to service programs through consultation on operating problems and through "translating" new and old social science knowledge that might be helpful to service personnel.

3. *In the long run, a broad approach to the social science aspects of public health problems will prove more useful than a specific, narrow focus.* Many of the public health programs have similar problems of public information, attitude, and behavior. Operational problems such as broken appointments, inability to reach the apathetic individual, and failure of clients to follow through on care or referral, can best be solved against a background of general

principles rather than treating each one as a special case. While a certain amount of social research may have to be devoted to the study of specific administrative or operational problems, the major focus of the social science program should be upon policy questions and administrative principles applicable to a wide range of problems.

4. *A social science program, to be meaningful, must be free to develop an inherently social science approach to public health problems.* As qualified professionals, the social scientists should be given the scope to develop their own program in the way their professional training indicates would prove most productive. This means accepting, and even encouraging, their desire to explore new areas of social science in public health and new social science approaches to the solution of old public health problems. In pursuing this policy, the social scientists will make use of their own unique methods of doing social research, qualitative as well as quantitative.

In operating terms, this means that social scientists are by and large used as social scientists and not as public health workers or researchers. It also means that the social scientist, like any other professional expert, should be consulted whenever a major problem of service or research involving social science principles arises.

In addition to serving as consultants to other programs, the professional staff of a social science program must be free, to a large extent, to define its own research problems and research methods. These problems, of course, should be directly related to the field of public health and to the current needs and interests of the health agency. But within these limits, the formulation of specific hypotheses and research designs should largely be the responsibility of the social science professional staff.

The goal of these policy statements is to create an environment in which social scientists can do their best work and make their greatest possible contribution to the field of public health. This environment will permit the social science staff to develop a feeling of identification with the goals of public health and a pride in its allegiance to the public health profession. It is intended to make possible a real integration of social scientists into a health agency founded on respect and consideration for each other's needs and values. It offers the only basis for a mutually satisfying working relationship.

NOTES TO CHAPTER VIII

1. Goode, William J., "Encroachment, Charlatanism, and the Emerging Profession: Psychology, Sociology, and Medicine," *American Sociological Review*, vol. 26, February, 1961, p. 902.
2. *Ibid.*, p. 906.
3. Russell Sage Foundation, *Annual Report, 1958–1959*, pp. 8–13.
4. Anderson, Odin W., and Milvoy S. Seacat, *The Behavioral Scientists and Research in the Health Field*. Health Information Foundation, Research Series 1, New York, May, 1957.
5. Freeman, Howard, Sol Levine, and Leo G. Reeder, "Present Status of Medical Sociology" in Freeman, Levine, and Reeder, editors, *Handbook of Medical Sociology*. Prentice-Hall, Inc., Englewood Cliffs, N. J., 1963, pp. 478–479.
6. Williams, Richard H., "The Strategy of Socio-Medical Research" in Freeman, Levine, and Reeder, editors, *op. cit.*, pp. 423–447.
7. Russell Sage Foundation, *op. cit.*, p. 12.
8. Foster, George, "Public Health and Behavioral Science: The Problems of Teamwork," *American Journal of Public Health*, vol. 51, September, 1961, p. 1288.
9. Anderson, Odin W., and Gerald Gordon, "Social Research in Respiratory Disease," *National Tuberculosis Association Bulletin*, February, 1961, p. 11.
10. Simon, Herbert, *Models of Man*. John Wiley and Sons, New York, 1957.
11. Hamovitch, Maurice B., "Utilization of Research Findings," *National Association of Social Work News*, vol. 1, November, 1960, pp. 19–21.
12. Social Science Research Council, *Annual Report, 1959–1960*, pp. 7–8.
13. State Charities Aid Association, *Proceedings* of an Invitational Conference on Social Research in the Development of Health and Welfare Agency Programs, April, 1961, pp. 9–10.
14. Gouldner, Alvin W., "Theoretical Requirements of the Applied Social Sciences," *American Sociological Review*, vol. 22, February, 1957, pp. 92–102.
15. Russell Sage Foundation, *Annual Report, 1959–1960*, pp. 8–9.

IX

PROSPECTS FOR THE FUTURE

CURRENT FORCES IN SOCIETY and developments in medicine are straining at the limitations imposed by the basic six or seven functions traditionally allocated to public health. Dwork now speaks of the four "A's"—aging, alcoholism, air pollution, and accident prevention; Ginzburg of the three "D's"—diet, drinking, and driving; someone else of the "R's"—radiation, rehabilitation, and recruitment. These are the public health problems of the future and the inevitable shift in emphasis from infectious agents to behavior of people is obvious. Stainbrook has this to say:

> Progressively, we are creating for ourselves an almost totally man-made physical, social, and cultural environment. Diseases and illness —accidents, air-pollution reactions, psychosocial stress responses, suicides, and health problems complicated or engendered by people-deficiency and by meaning-deficiency, faulty sick role experience, and inadequate, reluctant, or tardy access to the social and cultural resources for the prevention of disease and uneasiness, and for the prevention or retardation of its worsening . . . can be encompassed only by . . . intelligent organization.[1]

The externally imposed, mass disease prevention measures previously utilized in the control of infectious, communicable diseases are inappropriate for reducing the incidence of the chronic, degenerative diseases. Here the focus must be on the individual and his behavior, rather than upon noxious elements in his environment. Public health must now "motivate" the individual citizen to change his behavior and must secure community support for changes in the "social environment," rather than assuming its own control of the physical environment. It is difficult to overemphasize the extent to which public health has been forced to reorient itself in order effectively to counter this shift in the nature of disease and its prevention and treatment.

It might be profitable at this point to speculate on some new directions public health may take in the immediate future and to note how its entry into these new areas will affect the collaboration between the social sciences and public health. First, and perhaps of greatest importance, is the widespread concern over the prevalence of mental illness in America, which until recently had been focused primarily upon treatment and rehabilitation of patients suffering from the psychoses. There are, however, many indications that this narrow orientation is changing and that the shift in focus will strongly involve the field of public health. One aspect of this broadening of viewpoint is the recognition of the fact that a large segment of the population possesses undiagnosed mental illness and that much of it is psychoneurotic, rather than psychotic, in etiology and symptomatology. Recognition of the widespread incidence of nonorganic mental illness has necessitated a careful reappraisal of the facilities and methods available to cope with it. It is obvious that psychiatry does not have sufficient personnel to deal with this problem; it is also debatable whether it would be "socially functional" to provide psychotherapy for everyone suffering from emotional problems. Solution, or at least amelioration, of the problem appears to lie in several directions, all of which involve, in varying degrees, the collaboration of public health workers and social scientists.[2]

Moving from a "problem area" in which the legitimacy of public health's concern has been generally (albeit, grudgingly) acknowledged, let us examine the fruitfulness of public health activity in hitherto largely unexplored territory. We pose that the whole spectrum of the "social deviances," such as alcoholism, juvenile delinquency, narcotics addiction, suicide, and accidents, are problems appropriate (and uniquely amenable) to public health activity. As public health has increasingly shifted its focus (a) from the prevention of the organic, communicable diseases to the "social diseases," and (b) from the individual "host" and his "physical environment" to the individual *in* his primary groups and his "social environment," it has become increasingly aware that, ultimately, the various forms of social deviance would have to receive attention. It is not happenstance that many of them have recently been referred to as "social illnesses" or "socio-environmental health conditions."[3]

We believe that most of these "social health problems" will be ameliorated only when they are approached, as well as merely labeled, as "social illness," the etiology of which has its roots in the family, the neighborhood, the community, and the total society, and the treatment and prevention of which can come about only through control of these social forces. The public health profession, by virtue of its orientation, techniques, and specialties is uniquely suited to deal with these problems and, we predict, will increasingly come to assume responsibility for coping with them. The desirability of collaboration with the social sciences on these social and behavioral disorders is too obvious to require explication.

In an excellent analysis of the relationship between social science and organized health services, Roemer points out some of the many changes that are occurring in the field of medical care which have particular significance for public health and the social sciences.

> The provision of day-to-day medical care to persons of all income, the patterns of medical practice by solo practitioners in a century of highly specialized science, the social and professional conflicts involved in introducing public health innovations, the organization of services for the needy, correction of the serious national maldistribution of physicians and dentists, the tasks of rehabilitation of the disabled in the complex world of workmen's compensation and labor-management relations, the problems of effective services for the aged and chronic sick whose needs are greatest when their resources are lowest, meeting the needs of minority groups like Negroes and Indians, the coordination of hospitals and dozens of other autonomous agencies in a region—are these not problems par excellence for the sociologist and the anthropologist?
>
> And consider the enormous interest and value of comparative international social studies on varying patterns of preventive and curative health service organization in different countries and their relationships to differing social, political, economic, cultural, and historical settings.[4]

All of the aforementioned problems are basic to health and medical care—problems that are becoming increasingly urgent for the field of public health each day. The boundaries between prevention and treatment in the case of the chronic diseases and the behavioral and social disorders are so tenuous as to make it impossible for public health to avoid responsibility for medical care in these areas. As in all fields, there is a "cultural lag" between yesterday's traditional activities and today's needs. But there can be little doubt that these social-medical problems will become the target of tomorrow's public health programs.

Many of these health problems represent fundamental, complex, social processes not easily understood and still more difficult to control. In many instances, the only significant answers may involve drastic changes in the entire social organization of medical care. Is it any wonder that the sociologist today has no ready answer to offer the harassed public health practitioner! Public health takes some of its most difficult health problems—problems with which it is currently making little or no headway utilizing traditional methods and problems that reflect basic social or economic forces—and social science is asked to provide some easy solution involving only some minor administrative changes or simple psychological or social action. The field of public health must accept the responsibility for meeting these complex problems itself even if this means introducing fundamental changes in its current values, objectives, and modes of operation. To ask the social scientist for a quick "sociological solution" is to avoid this basic responsibility.

To say that a particular public health problem is closer to being a social problem than a medical problem, or that the carrying out of a public health program requires working with community forces is, however, not an answer to the problem; it is only an indication of the discipline that must be approached to formulate the research question. A common mistake of public health personnel is to label a problem as "sociological" and then to expect the answer to it to come forth automatically from the sociologist. This is no more true than to identify cancer as a medical problem and in so doing expect medical science to know the answer. Identification of a public health problem as sociological means that the discipline of sociology must be consulted in an effort to find an answer, not for a ready-made answer. It means that social research must become an adjunct of medical research in an attack upon the problem. And it also means that "social factors" become only hypothesized variables of unknown importance in the etiology of disease, to be challenged and disproved as well as proved. In their zeal to establish themselves, social scientists are likely to overlook the need for negative as well as positive evidence—to disprove, as well as prove, the relevance of social factors.

Although this appraisal has placed its major emphasis upon the contributions that sociology has to offer public health, this relationship is by no means a one-sided affair. Public health has much to contribute, in its turn, to sociology; substantively, methodologically, and theoretically. The sociologist conducting research on health problems is in a position not only to accumulate a great deal of significant data on the important but hitherto largely neglected social area of health and illness. He is also in a position to advance sociological knowledge generally about social organization, occupational structure, community action, individual behavior and communication, to mention only a few areas. Methodologically, social research in public health can greatly advance existing techniques of the sample survey, especially in relation to the panel or longitudinal study and the cross-cultural survey. The concern of epidemiological research with rigorous research designs involving adequate control groups and reliable measures of social factors can add greatly to our ability to study such factors. Specific areas such as the definition and measurement of social stress and social class are particularly promising. Finally, theoretically, social research in public health is greatly concerned with social process and social change as these affect health action, and research in these areas may be expected to advance current theory on such problems as individual and community decision-making processes, the relationship of perception to fact, of knowledge to attitude, and of attitude to behavior, the principles of communication and public opinion, practitioner-client roles, and structural-functional relationships in health organizations. The fact that these theoretical formulations must stand the test of practical application only increases the probability that they will be stated in researchable terms and be subject to verification.

We would like to end this rather enthusiastic report on the tremendous opportunities open to sociology in the field of public health on a note of realism. We have concentrated on those areas of public health activity particularly dependent upon community and individual behavior and cooperation. It has not been difficult to discover within current public health problems a growing need for a sociological approach in public health practice. However, to some extent, this has been an academic exercise. Theoretically, these social factors are of basic importance; practically, they are largely ignored and even scorned. The overwhelming proportion of public health practice, research, and teaching proceeds without the aid of social scientists or any systematic utilization of social science principles. The sociologist in the voluntary or public health agency, or in the school of public health or medicine, does not usually occupy any position of great prestige, or wield any substantial power. The "real" work of public health is still carried on by the traditional communicable disease programs and by environmental sanitation, and the "real" research still takes place in the laboratory. While social processes may lie at the heart of the matter, the arms and legs of public health continue to move without any appreciable direction from social scientists. Social science may be close to the core of public health, but it is far removed from the substance of everyday public health operations.

And perhaps this is as it should be. Certainly public health has much to do to consolidate its present gains using available techniques and knowledge. In the United States tuberculosis is down, but it is still high on the list of causes of death. Venereal disease has fallen, only to rise again. Poliomyelitis is on its way out, but a majority of people still require inoculation. More than 33 million people in rural areas still lack even the simplest type of excreta disposal facilities. Over five thousand communities, comprising from two to three million people, have no public water systems.

Rats continue to plague large metropolitan areas, as do water and air pollution. Each year finds new outbreaks of disease traceable to food, milk, or water.[5] These areas still constitute the bulk of the public health activities of the operating health agencies and the core of the curriculum of the schools of public health—and, as any sociologist who has worked in an operating health department or a school of public health can testify, to see the public health professional bring his technical knowledge and skills to bear upon these problems day after day can be a humbling experience.

It is toward the future that the sociologist must look for any significant role in public health work. The public health programs of tomorrow will find chronic disease control replacing communicable disease control, with a subsequent greater emphasis on social factors in etiology, treatment, and prevention. Mental illness and other disorders of social origin such as alcoholism, will rise to the top of the morbidity tables; in fact, they are already there. Special groups such as the aged and the disabled will demand and secure new public health services. Medical care, involving economic problems of health insurance and organizational problems in administrative medicine, will expand the treatment aspects of public health practice.

These are the public health problems of the future that will have to be met by a reallocation of financial and personnel resources, and it is in this reallocation that the sociologically trained public health professional or the public health trained social scientist may hope to move from his present position of hypothetical importance to an actual position of prestige and power in policy determination. And as this evolution from philosophy to practice takes place, so will the World Health Organization's definition of health included in its constitution become a living thing rather than a high ideal. "Health is a state of complete physical, mental and social well-being and not merely the absence of disease or infirmity."

NOTES TO CHAPTER IX

1. Stainbrook, Edward, "Health and Disease and the Changing Social and Cultural Environment of Man," *American Journal of Public Health*, vol. 51, July, 1961, p. 1011.
2. A large number of reports have recently appeared on mental health as a public health problem. A good summary statement is contained in Williams, Richard H., editor, *The Prevention of Disability in Mental Disorders*, Mental Health Monograph No. 1, Government Printing Office, Washington, 1962.
3. Suchman, Edward A., "The Addictive Disorders as Socio-Environment Health Problems" in Freeman, Howard, Sol Levine, and Leo G. Reeder, *Handbook of Medical Sociology*. Prentice-Hall, Inc., Englewood Cliffs, N. J., 1963, pp. 123–143.
4. Roemer, Milton I., "Social Science and Organized Health Services," *Human Organization*, vol. 18, October, 1959, p. 77.
5. Hanlon, John J., *Principles of Public Health Administration*. C. V. Mosby Co., St. Louis, 1960, pp. 680–681.